Androgen
Disorders
in Women

The Most Neglected
Hormone Problem

Theresa Cheung

Foreword by James W. Douglas, M.D.

Hunter House Inc., Publishers
P.O. Box 2914
Alameda CA 94501-0914

Library of Congress Cataloging-in-Publication Data

Francis-Cheung, Theresa.
Androgen disorders in women : the most neglected hormone problem /
by Theresa Cheung.
p. m.
Includes bibliographical references and index.
ISBN 0-89793-260-9 (cloth). – ISBN 0-89793-259-5 (paper)
1. Hyperandrogenism. 2. Hormones. 3. Women—Health and hygiene.
I. Title.
RG207.5.F73 1999
618.1—dc21   99-26580
CIP

Project credits

Cover Design: Big Fish	Book Design/Production: Andrea Reider
Copy Editor: Rosana Francescato	Developmental Editor: Priscilla Stuckey
Managing Editor: Wendy Low	Editorial Assistant: Jennifer Rader

Acquisitions Coordinator: Jeanne Brondino

Proofreader: Lee Rappold	Indexer: Kathy Talley-Jones
Publicity: Marisa Spatafore	Marketing Intern: Monique Portegies

Customer Service Manager: Christina Sverdrup,
Order Fulfillment: Joel Irons, A & A Quality Shipping Services
Publisher: Kiran S. Rana

Printed and Bound by Data Reproductions, Auburn Hills, MI

Manufactured in the United States of America

9 8 7 6 5 4 3   First Edition   01 02 03

Table of Contents

List of Illustrations

IMPORTANT NOTE

The material in this book is intended to provide a review of androgen disorders. Every effort has been made to provide accurate and dependable information. The contents of this book have been compiled through professional research and in consultation with medical professionals. However, you should be aware that professionals in the field may have differing opinions and change is always taking place. If any of the treatments described herein are used, they should be undertaken only under the guidance of a licensed health care practitioner. The author, editors, and publishers cannot be held responsible for any error, omission, professional disagreement, outdated material, or adverse outcomes that derive from the use of any of these treatments in a program of self-care or under the care of a licensed practitioner.

Foreword

by Dr. James W. Douglas

Androgen disorder is by far the most common female hormone disorder. It is also the most neglected and misunderstood. Close to 10 percent of all women have some form of androgen or "male" hormone problem, but there isn't much public awareness of the condition or its symptoms.

Symptoms of androgen disorder tend to appear gradually over a number of years and range from the mild to the serious. They include irregular periods, infertility, unexplained weight gain, fluid retention, fatigue, mood swings, acne beyond puberty, hair loss, and unwanted hair growth. These symptoms appear unrelated. They are easily overlooked, unrecognized, and undertreated. Many women don't seek treatment because they don't think anything is wrong. Others know something is wrong but feel embarrassed or guilty about seeking medical advice, because androgen disorders primarily affect appearance.

The symptoms of androgen disorder should not be dismissed or ignored. The problem carries with it potentially severe health risks, such as increased risk for diabetes, heart disease, and cancer. If you notice something unusual about your appearance or have persistent menstrual cycle irregularity, it is in your best interest to see a doctor. In most cases the condition can be treated safely and effectively.

There are so many misconceptions about the role male hormones play in women's bodies and the treatment of male hormone disorders in women. Few women know what androgens and androgen disorders are. A large number don't even know that they have male hormones. Many have not heard the term *polycystic ovary*.

There is a real need for more information and explanation in lay terms. *Androgen Disorders in Women: The Most Neglected Hormone Problem* fulfills that need. In a clear and accessible manner, this unique book encourages women to learn more about how their bodies work. It explains that men and women share the same hormones and that the presence of male hormones in a woman's body is not unnatural; in fact, the female body was designed to have male hormones as well as female hormones. It examines the part male hormones play in all stages of a woman's life, explores the causes and effects of androgen disorder, shows how the condition can affect a woman emotionally as well as physically, outlines the various treatment options available, and suggests ways women can help themselves.

Acknowledgments

My thanks to all the many people who helped provide information about androgen disorders for this book. In particular I would like to thank Dr. James Douglas, M.D., reproductive endocrinologist and infertility specialist at the Plano Medical Center in Texas, for permission to quote him and for his invaluable advice, comments, and help with research while I was writing this book. I would also like to thank all the women I talked to who have had some form of androgen disorder, for the insight they gave me into this complex condition. Their stories are in this book, with names and places changed to protect their privacy. They provided much of the incentive to write about a condition that has for too long been dismissed and ignored. I am also indebted to all the staff at Hunter House for their help, advice, encouragement, and insight throughout, as well as the fine developmental editing work of Dr. Priscilla Stuckey.

Thanks also to my brother, Terry, and for the support of friends and family. Finally, special gratitude to my husband, Ray, for his help with editing and for his patience, support, enthusiasm, and love while I completed this project.

Introduction
Why Read This Book?

C hances are you picked up this book because you have not been feeling well lately and want to know why. Perhaps you suffer from skin and hair problems, irregular periods, fatigue, and unexplained weight gain. You suspect that it might have something to do with your hormones but are not quite sure.

This book is for you. It will show you that you could be suffering from a medical condition, called *androgen disorder*, that can be easily explained and treated. It will show you that you are not alone. Simply knowing that there are millions of women out there like you will be reassuring. And I hope that by explaining to you what is going on in your body and by showing you how the symptoms can be treated effectively, I will encourage you to overcome any embarrassment or guilt you might feel, and seek medical advice.

There is, however, another side to this. It's tempting to blame hormones or glands for problems we don't want to take responsibility for:

I want to lose weight, but my glands are sluggish.

I used to feel sexy and energetic, but my glands aren't working so well any more.

I know I shouldn't have done that, but my hormones are all over the place.

Weight gain, mood swings, and loss of interest in sex can be the results of androgen imbalance, but they can also result from too much food, too little exercise, or a lack of challenge and discipline in our lives. Changes in hair condition and skin texture could be the result of a hormonal imbalance, but wrinkles and graying hair are a normal part of the aging process. It is important that we learn to distinguish between real hormonal dysfunction and other problems we might be having, rather than blaming our hormones to avoid facing issues in our lives. This book will help you determine whether hormonal problems are really causing any distressing physical problems you may have.

Perhaps you were attracted to this book because you wondered what the most neglected female hormone problem was. Maybe you were drawn to it because you were interested in the subject of male hormones in women, or you might just want to know more about your body. Whatever your reason for picking up this book, it will help you learn more about yourself and how your body functions.

It is important to understand how our bodies work. We often give very little thought to our bodies until something goes wrong. We all want to feel well. We all want to maintain the correct weight and have glowing skin and hair. We need to realize that this is possible only if our bodies are in a state of hormonal balance. Learning about hormones and how they affect our lives can help us recognize when there is an imbalance and know what we can do about it.

Women need to know their hormones better. We know hormones are produced by glands, and we know that hormones are responsible for certain bodily changes, but most of us lack a clear understanding of how important hormones are and what they do. The truth is that hormones coordinate every part of our lives throughout our entire life span. We can lead more productive, harmonious lives when we understand the vital role hormones play. If we can sort out the signs and symptoms of hormonal changes, we will gain a greater understanding of ourselves.

Despite what we were taught at school, male hormones, or androgens, are not just present in men, and estrogen and progesterone are not found only in women. Not only do men's bodies make female hormones, but women's bodies make male hormones. Men and women are not as different as we might think!

Male hormones are involved in female development. In order to have a real awareness and appreciation of our bodies, we need to fully respect the significance of both female and male hormones and the role they play in all stages of our lives. It is time that the whole subject of male hormones in women, and how they affect us, be given the attention it deserves. There has been so much focus on the so-called female hormones—estrogen and progesterone—but very little on the so-called male hormones in our bodies. This book will explain how vital a correct balance of androgens is for us to lead balanced, healthy, and happy lives.

Part 1

The Most Neglected Female Hormone Problem

1

Life with
Androgen Disorder

Why do I keep gaining weight, however hard I diet and exercise?

What are the health effects of missed periods?

I'm losing my hair, but I don't want to go bald. Is there anything I can do?

Are the cysts on my ovaries malignant?

How can my facial hair growth be linked to my irregular periods?

Aren't acne and bad skin caused by a poor diet?

What effect is this going to have on my sex life?

How much male hormone is normal for a woman?

The questions seem endless. You don't feel really sick, but you know something is wrong. You are not sure if you should see a doctor or not. Or perhaps you have gone to a doctor and been told you have androgen disorder. You want to find out more, but there is little information or guidance available for the layperson. You want to talk to friends and family, but the symptoms—missed periods, hair loss, acne, weight gain—are not easy to discuss. You feel embarrassed to admit you have a problem with "male" hormones. You feel isolated, cut off from other women. You don't feel as sexy or feminine as you once did. Maybe you're avoiding intimacy with your partner because you feel inhibited. You feel as if there is no one you can talk to. You feel alone in a world that lacks sympathy for women who have problems with their appearance, and one in which talk of menstrual problems is taboo.

You wonder why you are in this situation in the first place. Is it your fault? Is it a disease? Has your body forgotten how to be female? What is going on with those incomprehensible, unpredictable hormones of yours?

The term *androgen disorder* is little known. It sounds like some kind of rare disease, but this is definitely not the case. "You may be surprised to learn" writes Dr. Geoffrey Redmond in *The Good News About Women's Hormones* (p. 165) "that androgen disorders are the most common female hormone problem. . . . If you yourself do not have any androgenic problems you are certain to have a friend who does."

Week after week, the symptoms of androgen disorder are discussed in women's magazines, but the disorder itself is not named. Hardly an issue of some magazines goes by without an article related to acne, skin problems, weight problems, embarrassing facial and body hair, menstrual health, and so on. The anguish and confusion such symptoms cause women are vividly brought to life in these articles. Sound advice is given about stress reduction, diet, exercise, how to manage your weight, how to maintain glowing skin and hair. But these magazine articles often fail to mention hormonal problems as a crucial factor.

I'm really fed up. I never used to have a weight problem. Now I just look at food and I gain weight. I try to follow the advice

I read in books and magazines and see on the TV about diet and exercise and a healthy lifestyle. I work out most days, lead an active life, and eat as healthily as I can, but I don't seem to be able to lose the fifteen pounds I gained over the last year and a half.

I know there are more important things to worry about than my weight, but it's depressing me. My periods are also getting very unusual. Months will pass without one, and then I'll get a long and heavy bleed. My sister keeps telling me to see a doctor, but I wouldn't want to trouble my busy doctor with something trivial like weight gain and having irregular periods.

Nicola, age thirty-two

Nicola did finally go to see her doctor. She found out that she had androgen disorder. If you have androgen disorder you need to understand, like Nicola eventually did, that sometimes the symptoms won't just go away, despite every effort you make. Diet and lifestyle changes and self-discipline can, but don't always, work. You may need some kind of hormonal therapy.

Susan, age twenty-nine, also found help for her symptoms after seeing a doctor.

I used to think of myself as an energetic person, but last year everything changed when I stopped taking the Pill. I felt as if I was falling apart. I became anxious and moody; it was difficult to concentrate. I was depressed one moment, agitated the next, perpetually tired. Some days even walking up stairs was exhausting.

My doctor examined me and assured me I was not dying. He asked me when I had had my last period. I told him that I had not had one for six to seven months. He said I had secondary amenorrhea. I had never heard of the word and discovered that it is the medical term used to describe the absence of normal menstrual function in women before menopause.

I did not know whether to laugh or cry. Was the absence of menstruation some kind of precursor to menopause? Did I have a tumor?

The doctor said that probably a combination of many factors had caused the hormonal imbalance I was suffering from. He explained that many women experience amenorrhea at some point in their lives, especially when they are under stress. He asked me if I had been working too hard. He told me to try to find time to relax and to come back in a few months. He wanted me to go back on the Pill, but I told him that I was trying to get pregnant.

My husband assured me that everything would be all right. I appreciated his sympathy, but how could he understand what it felt like to be a woman without her natural rhythms? Having been married for a few years, I never knew what to say when friends kept asking when, or if, we were going to start a family. Amenorrhea was robbing me of the right to even chose whether to have a baby.

I returned in two months to see my doctor. My periods were still absent and my skin was breaking out in spots and blemishes. My hair lacked shine. I looked much older than twenty-nine. I exercised daily and watched my diet, but it was getting harder and harder to keep motivated. My husband was worried; he had never seen me so depressed. The weight was piling on.

This time I was referred to an endocrinologist. I was given a series of tests. She told me that I had an excess amount of male hormone circulating in my body. She said that this was interfering with my reproductive cycle and it was very likely that I had cysts on my ovaries. An examination confirmed this. It was explained that as long as I had this condition I would not be able to conceive. I was also told that the condition is very common. I suppose this was meant to make me feel better, but it did not really. I heard the word *cyst* and imagined the worst. All I thought was, if the condition is so common why have I never heard of it? Why did I have all that male hormone? It was embarrassing. Was I infertile?

Without really quite knowing what was going on, I agreed to have hormonal treatment. Within a few months my periods returned. The doctor tells me that as long as I take fertility drugs to make me ovulate, I have as good a chance as any woman in her early thirties of conceiving a child.

Susan's confusion and anxiety about her condition are not uncommon. There just isn't readily available information and advice about androgen disorder. This is astonishing, considering that as many as one in ten women in the United States suffers from the disorder.

If this is the case, why have so many of us not even heard the term *androgen disorder*? Why is there so little information and advice available?

One of the reasons may be that the symptoms of androgen disorder can be acutely embarrassing. Madeline, age thirty-three, made every effort to conceal her problem. She wouldn't think of seeing a doctor.

What I wouldn't give to be able to spend an afternoon without being terrified that someone at work might notice the hairs on my chin and upper lip!

It was when I left college that I first noticed the problem. It made life really difficult. My days were scheduled around when I would have to shave next. I would never leave the house without shaving. Even if I slept through the alarm clock, it was better to be late than not to shave. At work I would constantly check the state of my hair growth in the mirror. Every hour or so I'd get my hand mirror out and study my face. Sure enough, around two in the afternoon, the hairs began to resurface. Now things got complicated. I had to go to the ladies' room and shave. If anyone walked in I would hastily retreat into a stall and wait until they left. It would have been so embarrassing being caught shaving my face. I know every woman shaves her legs and underarms, but men get beards and mustaches and sideburns, not women! When work finished at around six or seven, I'd go straight home and shave again.

The problem caused tension in my relationship. My boyfriend never understood why I flew into a temper if he did not give me enough time to get ready before we went out. I needed time to shave. I toyed with the idea of telling him, but I never had the courage. I was sure he would think I was some kind of freak.

My facial hair growth became an obsession in the end. It constantly worried me. I spent thousands of dollars and many hours having electrolysis.

As well as the reluctance of many sufferers to bring attention to themselves, another reason for the neglect of a condition is the fact that symptoms range from the mild to the serious. Many women have mild symptoms, which they try to ignore or blame themselves for.

The symptoms seem so everyday: If you suffer from acne, you blame your diet. If you lose hair, you blame your stress level. If you have increased facial hair, you think it's because your mother had the same problem. If you put on weight, or if your complexion is always dull, you think it must be due to stress. If your mood is low or you lose interest in sex, you think it must just be a phase you are going through. If your periods are irregular, you hope things will just sort themselves out. You learn to deal with the discomfort. You get so used to adapting to the symptoms that you forget what feeling healthy is really like. You probably won't think of seeking treatment until really severe problems occur, or until you want to have a baby and find that you can't.

Basically you learn to live with the disorder. You accept problems with your appearance and less-than-perfect health as if they were the norm. Lucy, age thirty-nine, is typical:

> I used to worry about the irregularity of my menstrual cycle. I also wished I could lose some weight and have a clearer complexion. It never occurred to me to go to see a doctor to check if there was a problem with my hormones. I just thought every woman, except the lucky few, has problems with her periods, or her weight.

What is needed is greater awareness and understanding of androgen disorder. This is slowly beginning to happen. There is still a long way to go, but the importance of androgens in a woman's life is an area of research that is gradually developing. This research has lead to better treatment options than ever before from doctors and therapists alike. But despite this, there is still not enough advice for women. Doctors and sufferers themselves still neglect or dismiss the problem until it gets serious. Lauren, age thirty-five, is a case in point:

> I went to see my doctor two years ago. I had lovely, long, dark, curly hair, but I thought I was losing my hair. I had had much fuller hair a year or so before. The doctor could not see that there was a problem and assured me that my hair was fine. I remember bursting into tears. Why would nobody take me seriously? I knew I was losing hair. I remembered clearly the first time I first found a lot of hair in the bath after showering.
>
> In the months that followed I was constantly tearful and depressed. I thought that stress and depression were causing the problem, and I went into therapy. The therapy did not help.

As every day passed I seemed to be losing more and more hair. As every day passed I became more and more depressed. I didn't want to go out any more, because I feared people would notice. I started to wear scarves to disguise the problem. My once busy and active social life completely disintegrated.

Ten months later there was a definite thinning at the back of my head. Finally my doctor took me seriously.

Why do doctors pay so little attention to the condition and its symptoms?

Perhaps it has something to do with the medical profession's attitude toward female patients. We all know that men and women have different shapes, hormones, and psyches. It seems obvious that illnesses and medications will affect us differently. Yet while there has been a tremendous amount of new research into women's health in the last few years, medical schools have been slow to integrate the findings into their curriculums. Their approach is still male-centered. Women's bodies and particular hormonal makeup are underrepresented in medical textbooks. As a result, our hormonal problems are not given the attention they deserve. While the situation is slowly changing for the better—for example, we are being informed about the importance of a correct balance of estrogen and progesterone—the role androgens play in the female body is still overlooked.

Another reason the medical profession neglects the condition is that androgen disorders, in most cases, affect not only your health but your appearance too. Should medicine be concerned with appearance?

There is a strong case for arguing that it should. Sometimes changes in appearance can be harder to live with than many other illnesses. They are visual, whereas many illnesses can be concealed. Lauren was surprised at how much anxiety she felt at the thought of going bald. She was ashamed to admit that it affected her more than the death of her parents a few years earlier.

Problems like acne, hair loss, weight gain, and unwanted body hair growth are humiliating and disturbing. They should not be dismissed by doctors. Women with these problems feel not only embarrassment but also guilt over worrying about their appearance. Yet appearance is important, because it affects how you feel about yourself and how you function in your daily life. For example, a young woman training to be a teacher may suffer great anxiety that her increased facial hair will be noticed by the children she teaches and that she will be ridiculed. They might not notice, but how can she be sure? If her problem is treated, she will feel less anxiety.

Life is traumatic if you have an androgen disorder. Even if you know you are loved and accepted by those around you, there is always that insecurity: Perhaps people will notice your problem and hold it against you. Perhaps the problem will get worse. Perhaps there is something really wrong with you. Perhaps it is all your fault.

This book will try to take some of the distress out of androgen disorder by giving readers information and advice about the condition. After reading this book, if you think you have any of the symptoms of androgen disorder, the first thing to do is to see your doctor. He or she will tell you if hormonal imbalance is causing your symptoms.

If your condition is diagnosed as androgen disorder, you need to understand that hormonal imbalance is a medical condition. The symptoms can be treated and recovery is possible. It is also very important that you understand four very important points about androgen disorder:

1. The symptoms of androgen disorder tend to manifest gradually over many years, eventually resulting in severe problems. The condition is far easier for doctors to treat when symptoms are at the mild stage and the disorder has not fully established itself.

2. There are various degrees of androgen disorder. In some women, the symptoms are so slight—perhaps the odd missed period or bout of acne—that they won't really be aware of any problem. In other women, the symptoms are more severe: for example, persistent acne, or an excessive amount of facial hair from adolescence onward.

3. When symptoms of androgen disorder really do manifest suddenly, and there has been no prior history, you should see a doctor immediately. This is very dangerous. The most likely cause is a serious disease or tumor that needs urgent treatment.

4. Typically symptoms get severe when women reach their thirties. That is why medical textbooks usually state that women in their thirties are most prone to the disorder. This is not entirely accurate. You can have an androgen disorder at any age. Even if you notice it in your thirties, the disorder has been there since puberty but has been ignored because the symptoms seemed so mild. In the words of Dr. James Douglas, infertility specialist and endocrinologist at the Plano Medical center in Texas,

Androgen disorders can happen at any age. If you look at the older textbooks they discuss androgen disorders as a disease of women in their thirties. But if you question many women about the problem you find that they were manifesting very mild symptoms before this but never realized there was a problem. For example, their periods were never completely regular, but treatment was not sought until age thirty or so, when menses start getting really irregular. The problem, in the great majority of cases, just doesn't appear overnight.

Should symptoms suddenly appear, this causes the greatest concern. The symptoms could be related to an ovarian tumor, for instance. If a woman has always had totally regular periods and she suddenly starts growing facial hair and going bald, and her periods stop, urgent action is necessary.

The sudden-onset cases are rare. They are the most worrying and dangerous. Slow, gradual cases are the ones that we see all the time. But, just because symptoms are mild, this does not mean they should be ignored. It is very important, if a woman notices anything unusual about her appearance, or if she has noticeable cycle irregularity, that she go and see a doctor. Androgen disorders may be the cause, and, if this is the case, there may be serious health risks involved.

If you have androgenic problems, you need not feel alone. Women from all walks of life can experience the disorder, and there are ways to treat the condition and ways you can help yourself. The first step on the road to recovery is gaining awareness. The very fact that you are reading this book shows that you want to know more.

The following chapter will explain what hormones, androgens, and androgen disorders are. Part 2 will examine the many signs and symptoms of androgen disorder, and part 3 will focus on self-help and prevention and help you assess the various treatment options available from both conventional and alternative medicine.

Once the link has been made between your symptoms and your hormones, decisions will have to be made. Your doctor is likely to encourage you to take hormone replacement therapy. You will probably think this is the best thing to do, because the media heavily promotes hormonal replacement therapy as some kind of miracle cure. And indeed it can offer fast and often effective relief. When I wanted to have a baby, nothing but hormonal therapy and fertility treatment worked. I could have waited a few more years and tried other approaches, but I was already in my thirties and did not feel I had any time to waste.

For many women hormonal therapy is the answer, but for other women, it isn't. Even though some of their symptoms go away, they still don't feel that good. These women often feel better with a more gentle approach that encourages changes to diet and lifestyle. There is still so much for us to learn about hormones, and more and more women are finding that the symptoms of hormonal imbalance can be alleviated through nonhormonal therapy.

If you suffer from androgen disorder, you have to determine what works best for you. This book will encourage you to look at your own lifestyle and how it might in fact be contributing to problems with androgen levels, so that you can determine what the right course of treatment is for you. It will offer advice about both conventional and alternative medicine, as well as prevention and self-help tips related to diet, exercise, weight management, and stress reduction.

The symptoms of androgen disorder can be unpleasant and frustrating to live with. But the good news is that you don't have to live with them. If yours is like the great majority of cases, you can do something about the problem.

2

Hormones, Androgens, and Androgen Disorder

It took thousands of years for Western science to develop a theory about hormones. Although the Greeks preserved the story of Castrates, who lost his sexual potency, libido, muscle strength, and hair when his testes were removed, the idea that the testes secreted a substance necessary to the preservation of maleness was not to develop until much, much later.

As one century melted into another and knowledge of the human body increased, the major glands—the pituitary, thyroid, parathyroid, pancreas, adrenals, ovaries, and testes—were discovered. It took many years for their functions to become known, though, and for physicians to come to the conclusion that the endocrine glands discharged secretions into the bloodstream that influenced body function.

In the late eighteenth century, surgeon Percival Patt at St. Barts Hospital in London operated on a young woman to repair a hernia and inadvertently removed her ovaries. To the doctor's astonishment, her periods ceased and her breasts shrank. The connection between menstruation and a woman's ovaries and their secretions was made.

The word *hormone* first appears in a 1905 lecture by Ernest Henry Starling entitled "The Chemical Correlation of the Functions of the Body." Starling described hormones as circulating chemical messengers. He used the word *hormone* to refer to secretions from various organs in the body, such as the ovaries. These secretions circulate in the bloodstream as chemical messengers to regulate the metabolic needs of the whole body in order to maintain it in a good state of health. They set into motion events in the body that would otherwise not take place.

Over the next century and a half, the view developed that hormones are made in specific regions of the body, where they are released into the bloodstream and transported to target sites. It was believed that hormones coordinated the many physiological events that take place within complex organisms.

The hormonal system has turned out to be far more complex than this view anticipated. Hormones have been discovered all over the human body, as well as in less complex organisms. Many of their functions are still a mystery. Until the 1960s, scientists and doctors could name only a dozen or so hormones, but today we know of the existence of at least a few hundred. New discoveries are being made all the time. In fact, any substance that is produced by one cell and travels to another cell and affects how that cell functions can be called a hormone.

Each year, scientists and doctors learn more about hormones. Endocrinology, the branch of medicine and science that studies the endocrine system and hormones, is still developing. An endocrinologist is a doctor who specializes in hormonal disorders and disorders of the endocrine system.

Using hormonal treatment to improve the quality of our lives is at the forefront of modern medical research. More and more options are becoming available for using hormonal treatment. Human genes can actually be injected into bacteria to make them produce hormones, which can then be given to people who are suffering from hormonal imbalances. Diabetes, for instance, is treated in this way.

The area of hormonal research is incredibly exciting. One day, hormones may be produced to fight all kinds of diseases, such as AIDS and cancer. Since hormones affect how we feel, think, and behave, it is possible that destructive, violent behavior could be corrected with hormone treatments. Hormones affect how we age, so it is possible that in the future hormonal manipulation could ease the aging process itself. The possibilities are limitless. The scientific study of hormones is still in its infancy; there is much to discover.

HORMONES AND HORMONAL BALANCE

"I think of hormones as 'chemical communicators' or 'connectors'" writes Dr. Elizabeth Lee Vliet in *Screaming to Be Heard* (p. 35) "that carry messages to and from all organs of the body and serve to connect one organ's function with another organ's function to keep the body balanced and functioning optimally."

A correct balance of hormones is crucial for good health and normal adult development. Hormones regulate the body's functions and are necessary for life. The way you look, grow, feel, act and learn, the way your body digests food, grows hair, maintains its temperature, eliminates waste, and develops to adulthood—all these depend on hormones. Even the functions of some hormones themselves are regulated by other hormones.

So when hormone levels are normal we feel good, but when certain hormones levels are too high or too low, or when the body reacts to hormones in an unusual way, we won't feel so good.

If your body fails to produce certain hormones or produces them in either too great or too small amounts, this will lead to an imbalance, and you are likely to feel and look unhealthy. The giant, the dwarf, the vastly overweight woman, the man with bulging eyes, sweaty palms, and nervous tics, and the potbellied child who has the dried and crumpled skin of an old man are all tragic examples of what happens in extreme cases of hormonal imbalance.

Think of your hormones as members of an orchestra. Just as when one player is out of tune there is disharmony, an imbalance of one hormone will disrupt the entire endocrine system. Everything is so interconnected that if one hormone is not doing its job correctly, others will be affected. Hormones control life, sustaining activities like heart rate, respiration, digestion, immune response, and how we respond to stress. We need only minute quantities of these substances to keep our bodies in balance. Problems will occur if there is more or less than the normal level of a certain hormone in our body.

For instance, regular menstrual bleeding depends on a regular rise and fall in the hormones from the ovary and a delicate interaction between the brain and the reproductive organs at exactly the right time. It is an amazing piece of choreography, with complex moves that must be perfectly coordinated and balanced every month. If, however, for some reason the intricate balance is upset in any way, and the ovaries do not receive the right message at the right time, menstrual dysfunction is likely to occur. The same applies to other functions of the body that, like the reproductive cycle, are hormonally regulated. If the feedback system is disrupted, there will be problems.

THE SO-CALLED 'MALE' AND 'FEMALE' HORMONES

So far we have established that the endocrine system is regulated by its own hormones and that these hormones keep the body's systems functioning in perfect balance. If the balance is upset, the result is a progressive deterioration in health. This rule applies to both men and women. So it might seem logical to conclude that because men as well as women are governed by their hormones, men must be ruled by testosterone, the "male" hormone, and women by estrogen, the "female" hormone.

Not exactly . . .

It may come as a surprise to learn that not only is the "female" hormone, estrogen, present in men and actually made in the testes, but the "male" hormone, testosterone, is present in women and manufactured in the ovaries.

The 1990s have supposedly been a decade of greater aware-ness about hormones in women. But a 1997 study conducted at the Yale School of Medicine suggested otherwise. Although 98 percent of women believed estrogen to be a woman's natural hormone, and nearly 70 percent believed progesterone was too, only 46 percent thought that testosterone was a hormone that occurred in women. That means that over half of the women believed that only men produced testosterone.

Testosterone in a woman, estrogen in a man! We weren't taught about this in biology class. Our concept of male and female being absolute opposites is challenged by this.

It turns out that men and women are not as different as we would like to think. We both use the same hormones. To begin with, progesterone is considered to be a female hormone, but it is actually the chemical from which all the steroid hormones are made. Estrogen, a "female" hormone, and androgens, the "male" hormones, are both manufactured from progesterone. Women may have higher levels of progesterone than men, especially in the second half of our menstrual cycle, but neither sex could live without progesterone, as it is the source from which other hor-mones are made. Estrogen, the most "female" of all the hor-mones, is manufactured by the testes. The tiny amount of breast tissue that men have is a result of the estrogen in their bodies. When a man gets terribly overweight, his estrogen levels climb dramatically. Androgens, the "male" hormones, are active in women and manufactured in the ovaries and adrenals. They play an important role in female sexual development.

We share the same hormones. Estrogen belongs to a man's body and androgens are a natural part of a woman's body. The only difference is in the amount that we have. Generally, men have androgen levels about ten times as high as women's. From puberty on, testosterone blood levels in women need to be around 30 to 60 ng/dl. Men produce ten or twenty times as much, with blood levels running around 450 to 900 ng/dl. A high level of androgen in a woman would still be only three-tenths that of a man. So even when a woman has high levels of testosterone, her levels are far from being as high as those of a man.

In fact, we develop as women not because we have no androgens in our bodies, but because we have lower androgen levels in our bodies than men. Androgens as well as estrogen are the defining hormones in our lives at puberty. Our interest in sex is due to both the feminizing properties of estrogen and the libido power of testosterone.

Stranger even than the fact that a small amount of hormone of the opposite sex circulates in the blood of both men and women is the astonishingly tiny difference in the molecular structure of the masculinizing and feminizing hormones. They both belong to the class of hormones called *steroid hormones*, which have a common basic structure.

Figure 1 shows a picture of a steroid nucleus. Steroids are built around a molecular framework of four rings of carbon atoms. The carbon atoms in the rings are identified by a numbering system, and each represents what is called a "position." Each position is like a hook, and on this hook an additional carbon, hydrogen, and oxygen atom can be hung. Just a tiny change—the removal or addition of any of these additional carbons—can decide whether a hormone will regulate the body's water balance, cause hair to grow, or determine what sex a person will be. The difference between estrone (an estrogen) and testosterone is subtle. Figure 2 shows that the difference is just a shift in the position of oxygen and the hydroxil group. In this shifting the molecule can be either on its head or on its tail.

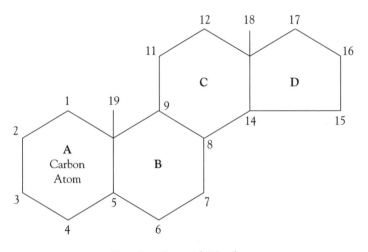

Fig. 1.   **Steroid Nucleus**

Incredible, isn't it, that there is so minute a difference between the molecular structure of male and female hormones!

Rigid classification of male and female hormones belongs to the past. The concept of female and male hormone dates back hundreds of years to an era when men and women were thought to be complete opposites. Modern medicine and science, however, have moved on. We can now reexamine the assumption that there are specific male and female hormones without fear of disapproval from church or state. We should stop regarding estrogen and progesterone as specifically female and androgens as specifically male. Our culture still tends to make sexual differences more absolute than they really are, even though the concept of androgyny is no longer so disturbing. It is time we realized that men and women are both human. In some ways, our bodies are more similar than they are different. Men, for instance, have a small amount of breast tissue, and women have a small amount of facial and body hair. Androgens belong to us, just as much as estrogen and progesterone belong to men. Having estrogen does not make a man

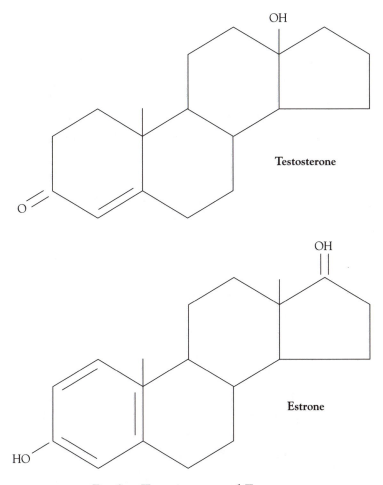

Fig. 2.   **Testosterone and Estrone**

less masculine, just as having androgens does not make a woman less feminine.

THE ENDOCRINE SYSTEM

Before taking a closer look at estrogen, progesterone, and androgens, let's review some basics about the functioning of hormones. What is just as remarkable as the functioning of our bodies is the fact that so many processes are identical in men and women.

The Glands

A gland is an organ that produces secretions. Exocrine glands secrete their substances outside the body; for example, saliva is excreted from the salivary glands. The endocrine glands secrete their substances inside the body directly into the bloodstream. The thyroid and ovaries are both examples of endocrine glands. The chemical compounds from these glands, known as hormones, regulate chemical reactions in our bodies via the circulatory system. The circulatory system consists of the heart, blood vessels, and blood and is a network of tubes within the body. It is the highway within which hormones travel in the body from their site of production to the tissues that respond to them.

In this book we will be chiefly concerned with the adrenal and ovarian glands, which produce androgens in women. Figure 3 illustrates where the endocrine glands are located in women and men. These include the hypothalamus, thyroid, parathyroid, pituitary, pancreas, pineal body, gonads (the sex glands), adrenals, and thymus. Men and women have exactly the same endocrine glands, except that women have ovaries and men have testes.

The Pituitary Gland

The pituitary, together with the hypothalamus, produces many of the hormones that control other glands (see figure 4). It is divided into two parts, or lobes. The front part is made of glandular tissue, and the back part is really an extension of the hypothalamus.

Until recently the pituitary gland, buried deep in the brain below the hypothalamus, was thought to be the master gland of the hormones, the gland that guides hormones to produce efficient body function. Today, the pituitary gland is no longer perceived as

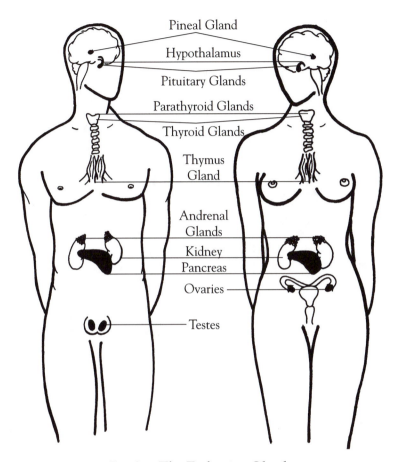

Fig. 3.   **The Endocrine Glands**

the ultimate regulator of the hormonal system. We know it responds to signals sent from the hypothalamus.

The Hypothalamus

The hypothalamus is the originator of a set of chemical signals that regulate numerous important functions in the body. As a center of control, it sorts out the mysterious messages from the brain and translates them into the language of hormones. It is a small region of the brain located just above the pituitary gland. It stands

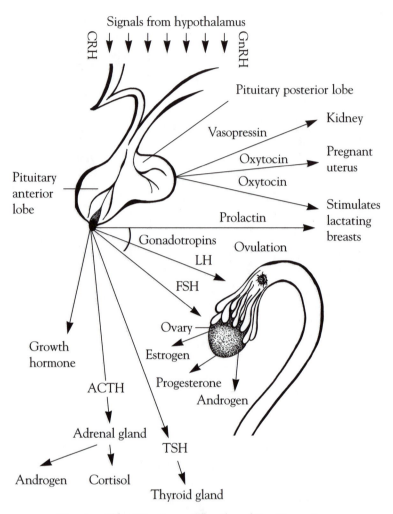

Fig. 4. **The Pituitary Gland and Its Functions**

at the apex of the body's hormone network and is in charge of integrating signals coming from there to the rest of the body.

For instance, gonadotropin-releasing hormone (GnRH) from the hypothalamus in women causes the pituitary gland to release luteinizing hormone (LH) and follicle-stimulating hormone (FSH), which stimulate estrogen, progesterone, and androgen production in the ovaries. Corticotropin-releasing hormone (CRH) from the hypothalamus stimulates the release of ACTH (corticotropin) from the pituitary, which causes the adrenal glands to produce androgens and cortisol.

The hypothalamus is often thought of as the hormonal control center. It might, however, be more accurate to say that, if there is a master gland at all, it is not the hypothalamus or the pituitary but the brain itself. In the brain, signals are received and integrated into the hypothalamus, which in turn manufactures chemical messengers that stimulate the pituitary and other glands in the body to produce hormones.

THE GLANDS THAT PRODUCE ANDROGENS IN WOMEN

Androgen hormones in women are manufactured in the adrenal and ovarian glands. The adrenal and ovarian glands respond to signals sent from the hypothalamus and pituitary and the brain.

The Adrenal Gland

Weighing just a few grams, the two adrenal glands are located above the kidneys; the left gland is longer than the right. Their importance in the maintenance of life was not known until the middle of the nineteenth century, when Thomas Addison discovered that profound debility resulted from disease of the adrenals. Each gland is divided into two parts: the inner core is called the *medulla* and the outer shell is called the *cortex*. The adrenal cortex produces a group of hormones commonly referred to as *steroids*. Steroids control the body's fluid balance, regulate the metabolism of blood sugar, maintain blood pressure, and enable the body to respond to stress. The sex hormones, estrogen and testosterone, are also secreted by the cortex.

The Ovaries

The ovaries lie just below the fallopian tubes on each side of the uterus. They are oblong and pearl-shaped. Ovaries produce eggs about once a month, which have the potential to become fertilized when they are released into the fallopian tubes. Ovaries also produce hormones—including estrogen and progesterone and androgen—throughout the life cycle, but the amount produced will vary depending upon a woman's age. At one time it was thought that androgen was produced only in the adrenal glands, but in the last few decades research has established that both pre- and postmenopausal ovaries produce androgen.

The production of the most powerful androgen, testosterone, in the ovaries corresponds to the production of testosterone in the adrenals. Most of this is converted to estrogen, but not all. Enough testosterone remains unconverted to account for one-quarter of our testosterone. Another quarter is produced in the adrenals. The rest is produced by tissues in different parts of the body, including the liver, skin, and hair, but these tissues manufacture testosterone from hormones that were made in either the ovaries or the adrenals. So, indirectly or directly, the ovaries and adrenals create all the androgens in our bodies.

THE SEX HORMONES

We will now take a closer look at the hormones that are responsible for sex characteristics, especially estrogen and the androgens.

Estrogen

Estrogen (from the Greek word meaning to produce desire or madness) is commonly regarded as the female sex hormone, although it is present in men too. It influences the thickness of the uterine lining and is responsible for many female characteristics. Breast

growth and development, external female genitalia, vaginal lin-
ings, and secretions and deposits of body fat are all dependent on
estrogen. The hormone also has a wider effect on the whole body,
influencing blood proteins, fats, and the production of blood vessels and bones. Levels of estrogen rise and fall at the command of
the pituitary gland, and the fluctuations usually follow a regular
pattern that coincides with stages of the menstrual cycle.

The effect of an imbalance of the "female" hormones estrogen
and progesterone in women is well documented. The risks of estrogen deficiency, especially, have now become common knowledge.
Television commercials, advertisement campaigns, and best-selling
books are devoted to the subject in an attempt to increase awareness. For instance, the Wyeth-Ayerst Women's Health Research
Institute—for the discovery and development of medicines that
help women lead healthier lives—produced in December 1997 an
ad campaign in national magazines and publications. The advertisement was striking. It showed a faceless, naked female body with
the brain, heart, and reproductive organs highlighted. Arrows
pointed to the sex organs, eyes, teeth, bone, and colon. Beside each
arrow there was a brief factual warning about how estrogen deficiency will affect these vital organs. Reduction in breast size, dry
skin, poor vision, tooth and hair loss, vaginal dryness, frequent
urination, risk of colon cancer, muddled thinking, hot flashes,
osteoporosis, and heart disease were just some of the symptoms
mentioned. The message was "Talk to your doctor," because problems with estrogen deficiency will affect the entire body.

It is a positive development, in contrast to the previous male-
centered approach to health issues, that so much information and
advice is now readily available about problems that are uniquely
female. There was a time when the distressing physical and emotional symptoms connected with estrogen deficiency were
thought to be "all in the mind"! Thankfully, we have come a long
way since then. Doctors are aware of the risks of estrogen and

progesterone imbalance, and we are being educated and informed about these. However, we are still not being informed about the important role androgens play in our lives.

Androgens

Androgens (from the Greek *andros*, meaning masculine) are nineteen carbon steroid hormones derived from cholesterol. They are secreted by the adrenal cortex and the ovaries. Androgens may also be derived from the conversion of other androgens by tissues such as the muscles and the skin. Androgens circulating in the body include testosterone (T), dihydrotestosterone (DHT), androstenedione (A4), dehydroepiandrosterone (DHEA), and dehydroepiandrosterone sulfate (DHEAS).

Testosterone

> Testosterone. Isn't that the hormone I shouldn't have too much of? It will make me grow a beard, won't it?
>
> It will make my voice deepen and make me get big muscles, I think.
>
> Testosterone. That's not good for me. I mean, I don't want to start looking like a man.

Of all the androgens, testosterone is the one everybody thinks they know something about. Unfortunately, much of what we think we know is wrong. Let's start by trying to clarify things a little and telling the truth about testosterone in women.

Testosterone is manufactured in our ovaries and adrenal glands; there is debate among medical researchers about which of these glands is our main source of testosterone. Other androgens, like DHEA, are just not as powerful as testosterone, and even when they are present in large amounts, they are used by the body to make more testosterone. And testosterone controls the behavior of other androgens. All this makes testosterone the most important and powerful androgen. Almost all the testosterone in a woman's body (99 percent) circulates in the blood, bound to proteins, of which the most important is sex hormone binding globulin (SHBG). There is always a small amount of remaining unbound testosterone, known as free testosterone, which is free to act on body tissues. Usually a mere 1 percent of all testosterone in the body is free, but in women with androgen excess this level can be as high as 2 percent.

Both bound and free testosterone affect the body. Free testosterone does so more directly, because it can move to tissues faster. But bound testosterone is gradually released by SHBG to become free testosterone, which also finds its way out of the blood and into the skin and hair. If either free or bound testosterone is high, there is androgen excess in the body.

How Does Testosterone Work?

First, testosterone is released from the adrenals or ovaries and travels in the bloodstream. Since blood travels everywhere in the body, testosterone can reach every organ. Once it reaches a tissue, the blood transports testosterone to the cells. The testosterone attaches to a cell at special holding areas called *receptors*. The cells of some tissues, such as those of the genital areas, have more testosterone receptors than others. As we grow older, our numbers of testosterone receptors diminish.

Once the testosterone is attached, the cell draws it into the cell body (see figure 5). The testosterone is then transported to the command center of the cell, the nucleus. The nucleus activates the body's genes to carry out the hormone's function.

DHEA

DHEA and DHEAS are the most abundant androgens secreted from the adrenal gland. Their function is not fully known, but they seem to be important in sustaining the metabolic balance of

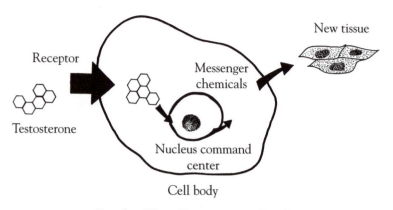

Fig. 5. **How Testosterone Works**

youth and keeping the immune system strong. About age thirty the body's production of DHEA starts to decline.

Research has shown that DHEA has many functions related to health and longevity. Among other things, it helps generate the sex hormones estrogen and testosterone, decreases the percentage of body fat, stimulates bone deposition, thereby preventing osteoporosis, and increases muscles mass. AS DHEA levels diminish with age, the structures and systems of the body may decline with it, making the body more vulnerable to age-related diseases and autoimmune conditions such as lupus and Reynaud's.

You can now do urine tests for DHEA (see Resources section), and DHEA supplements are available in nonprescription-strength pills and capsules and in higher-dosage prescription-strength pills and capsules. Many people who take them report increased energy and an enhanced sense of well-being.

There is as yet no conclusive research about the benefits of DHEA supplementation. We do know it can have undesirable side effects. The wrong dose of DHEA can suppress the body's natural ability to synthesize the hormone and lead to liver damage. If you do decide to take it, seek expert medical advice.

Maintaining the Androgen Balance

It is the androgens in men that produce masculinization—that is, a deeper voice, body hair, and so on. Even when a man has much higher levels than normal, ill effects are unusual. But in a woman, even a small change in normal androgen levels leads to detectable physical changes, such as acne or hair growth.

A woman's body continually produces a small but essential amount of androgen hormone. In order for us to feel well it is necessary to maintain this level of androgen. If your androgen levels fall below the required amount, you may feel tired, lack energy, and perhaps even experience a loss of sexual desire. You may also notice that your muscles lose tone, that your hair lacks shine and your skin its glow, and that your periods become irregular. Your mood may also be a little flat. Testosterone deficiency can also affect red blood cell production and the level of calcium in the bones, leading to osteoporosis. Loss of muscle tone in the bladder will also cause urinary incontinence. If, on the other hand, androgen levels rise above the crucial point, you could develop menstrual irregularity, acne, increased facial hair, scalp hair loss, and maybe even a lower voice. The symptoms of excessive testosterone are referred to as *virilizing effects.*

All women are very sensitive to small amounts of testosterone, so even a small increase in our normal level can make an incredible difference in how we feel. A normal amount of testosterone in a healthy woman is around 1.25 milligrams a day. Total blood levels are from 20 to 80 nanograms per deciliter. This is the level that treatment for androgen disorder or androgen deficiency will try to achieve. But what is normal for you may not be normal for someone else. To feel really healthy it is necessary to maintain the tiny, but crucial, level of testosterone hormone that is unique to you and you alone.

The Role of Androgen in Women

As far as those of us with androgen disorder are concerned, androgens are responsible for unattractive, unfeminine bodily characteristics such as facial hair, oily skin, and muscle buildup. When there is an imbalance of androgen hormone, there certainly will be unpleasant symptoms, and these will be discussed in more detail in part 2, but it is important to understand that when androgen levels are in balance these hormones have many benefits for women. Let's take a brief look at the role they play in female development.

Birth and Childhood

Incredible as it may seem, sex determination in the womb is not complex and dramatic. The process that determines the difference between a man and a woman takes only a few days and involves a few thousand cells. It also requires the active intervention of estrogen and androgen.

The old story, taught for the past fifty years, was that prenatal development tended toward the female. It was believed that a fetus would remain female unless there was an active intervention of androgens, which would make the fetus male. Recent research is proving that the old story of the female fetus could be part of an active-male, passive-female stereotype that regarded female development as a passive process and male development as active. According to Anne Fausto-Sterling, author of *Myths of Gender*, research shows that it takes the intervention of estrogen to nudge the fetus toward the female, just as it takes the intervention of testosterone to nudge the fetus toward the male. This is exciting, because it shows that neither hormone is passive.

During the embryonic period (weeks three to eight of human development), female fetuses cannot be distinguished from male fetuses in their outward appearance. During early fetal development (from the ninth week), outward differences between the sexes begin to take shape. The differentiation of male and female sex organs depends on the genetic makeup of the fetus and the complex interplay between hormones and tissues in the developing fetus. This interplay of factors results in the development of male and female reproductive characteristics by the end of the third month, with the penis in the male and the clitoris in the female developing from the same embryonic tissues. Likewise, the scrotum in the male is of the same evolutionary origin as the labia in the female.

Around the time of birth, the hypothalamus in the brain becomes very sensitive to the sex hormones estrogen, androgen, and progesterone, and only tiny amounts are produced. Babies will have enough hormone to differentiate their sex, but not enough to mature sexually.

From birth to puberty, girls and boys will have about the same low levels of testosterone and estrogen, which promote growth after birth. Everything springs to life when the hypothalamus begins to send signals to the endocrine glands at puberty. Now, along with thyroid hormone, growth hormone, and cortisol, androgen and estrogen once again control growth and sexual development.

Puberty

With the approach of puberty, the hypothalamus prompts the ovaries and the adrenal glands to start producing larger amounts of the sex hormones estrogen and androgen. Without estrogen and androgen to bring about the changes at puberty, there would be no reproductive life. Our species would end, stifled by a deadly loss of sex characteristics and fertility.

Throughout puberty, androgen and estrogen influence the development of secondary sex characteristics. Estrogen controls breast development, changes in the vagina and its excretions, and enlargement of the external glands. Androgens, which are secreted by the ovaries and the adrenal glands, control the growth of pubic and auxiliary hair, stimulate linear growth, weight gain, and the secretion of growth hormone by the pituitary, and speed up the maturation of the bones. When bones are mature a person cannot grow anymore, so androgens could well determine when growth ends.

Just as the beginning of menstruation is called *menarche*, the beginning of adrenal production of androgens is called *adrenarche*. Puberty is initiated by the production of androgen and estrogen, which together "kick start" sexual maturity. Girls start to produce testosterone in the adrenal glands much earlier than boys do, explaining why most of us mature earlier than boys at puberty.

At the end of puberty, bones mature and height becomes fixed. This happens at about age sixteen to seventeen in girls, and eighteen to nineteen in boys. After this the hormones that affect growth, such as androgen, still operate in the body and influence metabolism, as well as the growth of muscles and other body tissues.

The physical changes of puberty are also accompanied by emotional conflicts and upheavals, some of which are hormonally triggered. Sudden unpredictable mood swings in adolescents could be due to the surges in certain hormones taking place in the body. Adolescents often find it hard to explain why they feel a certain way, why they are behaving as they do. This may well be the truth: adolescents can be at the mercy of their hormones—in particular, androgen and estrogen.

The Benefits of Androgens to Women

We know that our bodies make androgens, but at much lower levels than men. We know also that there are many mistaken notions about androgens. They will not turn us into men and they are not bad for us; in fact, we need low levels of androgens to stay healthy.

Many doctors and researchers now believe that testosterone acts on the brain to stimulate sexual interest and may even affect sensitivity to sexual stimulation and orgasmic ability in both sexes. It is also believed that the nipples, clitoris, and vagina have testosterone receptors that can make you feel more sexual. For women to have an optimal sex drive, testosterone blood levels need to be at the required level. Most experts believe we need both estrogen and testosterone to feel sexual desire and to enjoy sex.

As well as possibly playing a role in libido, androgens affect our skin, hair, and menstrual cycle. They could influence our mood and cognition, too. Some researchers even go so far as to claim that there are testosterone receptors in the brain that establish the neurochemical basis for falling in love.

In addition, testosterone and the other androgens affect every tissue in our body in some way. Androgens are called anabolic steroids, meaning they make things grow and create muscle mass. Their effects include anabolic reactions (tissue build-up), body growth, nitrogen retention, and muscular development. Testosterone plays a crucial role in keeping the cells of the body functioning efficiently, making the best of nourishment for growth and maintenance, and particularly contributing to the health of bones and muscles. It acts on muscles, the liver, and blood vessels. Throughout our lives it helps maintain our muscle tissues, and because muscles are fat burners, androgens are important for weight management. Testosterone also helps build bone. This is one of the most important roles for testosterone in women, especially as we get older and lose the effects of estrogen in maintaining bone density. In the words of Dr. Susan Rako, a Newtonville, Massachusetts, psychiatrist (*Hormone of Desire*, p. 44), "With adequate testosterone, we have the maximal opportunity to experience our body's innate vital energy and sense of well-being." Rako goes on to say that physiologists believe that without effective testosterone the body develops a "catabolic state," in which tissues decline and muscle tone, vital energy, and a sense of well-being are lost.

If we are to believe such reports, it would seem that testosterone adds zest to our lives.

The Reproductive Cycle

Androgens are also part of the hormonal team that regulates the menstrual cycle. They fluctuate throughout the menstrual cycle, with peak levels at ovulation. When androgens, along with estrogen and progesterone, are at the optimal level, the menstrual cycle will be regular. But if androgen levels are elevated, the menstrual cycle will be disrupted.

Irregular periods should never be ignored. Your body is meant to have regular periods; that's how it was designed. If you notice that you have been skipping periods, or that your periods are absent, you should seek medical advice and have your androgen levels checked. We will discuss menstrual irregularities in chapter 4.

Perimenopause, Menopause, and Beyond

As we age, so do our endocrine glands, the sources of our male hormones. The changes are gradual and take place over several years. We do not suddenly realize one day that we are in menopause. Leading up to it for more than a decade or more are a wide variety of hormonal changes that cause physical and psychological changes.

Between the ages of thirty to fifty we enter the phase called the perimenopausal years, during which ovarian production of estrogen and progesterone begins to decline in preparation for menopause, when ovulation stops altogether. Androgen levels also begin to decline. Many functions are affected by these gradual hormonal changes, including sleep; memory; energy level; body fat distribution; functioning of the circularly system, digestive tract, and bladder; bone metabolism; and sexual function.

Menopause usually occurs between the age of forty-five and fifty-five, but it can occur in a woman's late thirties or even earlier.

For a variety of reasons, in the later years of the reproductive cycle, hormonal signals sent from the pituitary gland to the ovaries cease to be as effective, and the balance of hormones necessary to sustain the menstrual cycle begins to decline. Without hormonal support, the ovaries eventually cease to function and the uterine lining stops shedding every month in menstruation. The transition that we call menopause has occurred. For the rest of her life a woman will not have a menstrual period, and she will no longer be able to bear children. Frequently, this stage in life is accompanied by physical symptoms, as the body adjusts to the hormonal shifts taking place. These include profuse sweating, mood shifts, and changes in appetite and sleep patterns.

From our twenties to our forties the amount of testosterone in our body declines by up to 50 percent. After menopause we lose 66 percent or more of estrogen production and an additional 30 to 50 percent of androgen production. Many women do not notice this happening, but for some women testosterone decrease is accompanied by unpleasant side effects. Declining testosterone levels at menopause may account for the lack of vital energy reported by many menopausal women. It could also explain a loss of sexual desire, a lack of sensitivity in the nipples and genitalia, sparse pubic hair, difficulty concentrating, weakening of muscle tone, and the higher risk of osteoporosis.

The testosterone drop-off at menopause causes symptoms of varying degrees in different women. Rako lists decreased sexual desire, decreased sensitivity to sexual stimulation, and diminished capacity for orgasm (*The Hormone of Desire*, pp. 54 ff.). Other experts believe that a decline in testosterone affects mood and behavior. According to Dr. Michael J. Rosenberg, president of Health Decisions, Inc., a Chapel Hill, North Carolina, research group, symptoms include depression, anxiety, moodiness, insomnia, fatigue, and difficulty concentrating.

Prescribing testosterone at menopause is still somewhat controversial. Many doctors assert vigorously that lack of interest in sex is almost never due to hormones. The whole area still needs to be clarified, but there is growing evidence that testosterone has benefits to women.

Hormonal shifts, such as the decline in androgen level at menopause, will affect every woman differently, but the key to a successful transition lies in a woman's attitude toward menopause. We are not helped here by the fact that much of what is said about menopause tends to cast a negative light on the experience. Many of us still find it hard to deny that what is referred to as the "change of life" seems more like the end of life. Stereotypical images flash through our minds of bitter, vindictive, jealous, neurotic, and impossible old women suffering psychological disorders, with strange symptoms such as hot flashes, depression, and irritable behavior. Consciously or unconsciously, we are apprehensive about menopause and wonder how we will cope. We regard it not as a natural process but as part of aging and declining. When the reproductive organs start to atrophy, it is easy to feel it will not be long before the rest of us does, too.

The idea that menopause means getting old and no longer having a role to fulfill in society should be obsolete due to changes in cultural attitudes and advances in medical research. In today's society a woman's importance is no longer measured and defined solely in terms of childbearing, and we know that the fact that a woman cannot bear children anymore does not mean she cannot be sexual. Important medical research has demonstrated that the uncomfortable feelings that accompany menopause are not due to decline, atrophy, or decay but are caused by hormonal factors. The common physical discomforts of menopause, both sexual and emotional, result indirectly or directly from a lack of estrogen, progesterone, or androgen. Treatment can be sought to ease these discomforts. More and more is also being discovered about how a proper diet, regular exercise, and alternative therapies can alleviate the symptoms of hormonal imbalance at perimenopause for those who want to avoid hormonal therapy.

Crucial also is your attitude toward the bodily changes taking place. If you can understand what is going on with your hormones and successfully negotiate your way through our society's negative attitudes about menopause, you will discover that it can be a positive experience. Menopause comes with dramatic and often difficult changes to deal with, physically, emotionally, and mentally, but, as Joan Borysenko writes in her insightful study *A Woman's Book of Life*, menopause can be seen as "a second puberty, an initiation into what can be the most powerful, exciting, and fulfilling half of a woman's life" (pp. 140 ff.). We can find fulfillment both personally and socially. We can engage in both sexual and nonsexual relationships that are mutually satisfying. In freeing us from the reproductive cycle, this stage in life offers us the opportunity to fully understand ourselves, our sexuality, and what we have to contribute to the world.

ANDROGEN DISORDER

"Androgens are the forgotten hormone in a woman's body, only thought of when they cause a problem, which unfortunately they often do," writes Dr. Geoffrey Redmond in *Women's Hormones* (p. 38).

Androgen decline at menopause is a perfectly natural part of the aging process. It should not be confused with androgen disorder, which occurs when the mixture of hormones released into the blood from the ovaries and the adrenal gland is unnaturally high or too low for your age, or when there are problems with how the body reacts to androgen.

Androgen disorder is a syndrome, but it is not often diagnosed as such. All too often too much attention is paid to its symptoms, such as acne, weight gain, or thinning hair, and the underlying problem of an imbalance of androgen hormone is not addressed.

In the words of Tori Hudson, from the *Women's Health Update* on the Web, "What is in fact a syndrome is often viewed segmentally; we treat the acne or the alopecia [hair loss] but do not tie it together with the menstrual irregularity, or we see the infertility but do not associate it with the adolescent acne, or we see the glucose intolerance problems but do not see it as related to the excess hair on the upper lip" ("Androgens and Women's Health," http://www.thorne.com/townsend/mar/wns_update.html.).

Symptoms of Androgen Disorder

The symptoms of androgen disorder fall into three main groups: changes in appearance, abnormal menstrual patterns, and metabolic and systemic disorders. These symptoms will be examined in more detail in part 2.

According to Dr. James Douglas,

> The most common symptoms are cycle irregularity, acne beyond puberty, hair in places where women wouldn't want hair, and weight gain. These are symptoms that one wouldn't necessarily connect with a hormonal disorder. They are easy to underestimate, because they are multiple symptoms. You might not think they are all connected to the one cause. A woman would not connect irregular periods to her acne. She would not know that the hair on her chin is connected to her ovaries.
>
> It's interesting when a woman comes in to see me about her irregular periods. I discuss polycystic ovary and the ovaries making too much testosterone. I tell her that on top of having irregular periods and not being able to get pregnant, she probably has excess hair and acne and can't lose weight, when she eats the same calories as every one else. She often looks surprised and asks me how I know all that, as I have not even run any blood tests and no doctor has told her this before. I tell her I know because these are the symptoms of polycystic ovary, when the body overproduces androgens. Perhaps when she went to a doctor before there was no time

to explain and she was simply given the birth control pill to regulate her periods.

When there is androgen disorder, every woman will have an individual response to the problem. Not everyone will have all the symptoms in excess. You have mild and severe versions. You have women who don't have excessive hair or acne but who have irregular cycles. These women have a mild condition. Then there are women with severe problems who shave every day, have weight they can't lose, and have terrible acne. Some women may also have just one symptom— hair growth for instance, or acne—but most tend to have a mild version of all the symptoms.

The Mysteries and Complexities of Androgen Disorder

Androgen disorder is an extremely complex and mysterious condition. There is often no one simple explanation for it, and a combination of factors may be involved. We don't really know what causes it. Some doctors suggest clinically defined causes, and others think emotional and psychological factors, poor diet, and stress play a part. Some of the possible causes will be outlined in part 2, "The Signs and Symptoms of Androgen Disorder."

Not only don't we really know what causes androgen disorder, but we also can't be sure how it will manifest in each woman, because each case is different. Androgen level elevations do not necessarily have obvious clinical manifestations, and vice versa. For instance, one woman may have an increase in androgen production, plasma concentration, and metabolic clearance, while another will have an increase in androgen and plasma concentration but no metabolic problems, and yet another may have androgen excess and metabolic problems but normal plasma concentrations. And each woman reacts differently to androgen. Some will react to high levels, while others are sensitive to normal androgen levels. Some will get acne, some won't, some will have irregular periods and some won't, and so on.

In short, the symptoms of androgen disorder will be unique to each woman. The condition is complex and unpredictable. To help you recognize the many signs and symptoms of the condition, the next section of this book will examine them in more detail.

Remember that the symptoms of androgen disorder can be easily misunderstood and misdiagnosed. Say you notice a slight increase in facial hair. Perhaps you have been steadily gaining weight and feeling tired lately. Maybe your hair is thinning, or your complexion is dull. Has that old acne problem returned? Have your periods become irregular or stopped altogether?

Surely, you may think, there is nothing to worry about. Isn't every woman at times concerned about the condition of her skin and hair? What woman isn't worried about her weight? And aren't irregular periods and PMS just facts of life?

There certainly is something to worry about! When you don't feel as healthy as you know you could feel, there is reason for concern. Your body is trying to tell you something. It wouldn't be wise to ignore these symptoms, however vague they may seem. They are your body's way of alerting you to the fact that something is wrong. There could be a problem with your androgen levels, and if this is the case, you must seek treatment. Left untreated, androgen disorder carries with it severe health risks.

Part 2

The Signs and Symptoms
of Androgen Disorder

3

Changes in Appearance

I'm so tired. Tired of shaving every day. Tired of washing my skin over and over again. Tired of washing my hair twice a day. But most of all I'm tired of worrying about what others will think.

Mary, age thirty-one

My mom always said I'd grow out of my acne. Well, I'm thirty-two and still plagued with sore skin, redness, and spots. It's embarrassing. I'm not a teenager anymore. Why have I got this problem? What I wouldn't give to have a clear complexion.

Jennifer, age thirty-five

My husband tells me that the dark hair on my legs and chest doesn't bother him. He says that he thinks it makes me sexy. Why doesn't that make me feel better? Why do the disapproving glances I get from other women bother me so?

Cynthia, age forty-one

ndrogen disorder will primarily affect your appearance. Most noticeable will be the effect it has on your hair and your skin. When symptoms manifest in this way, they are often misdiagnosed and misunderstood. You shave or pluck. You buy expensive skin creams. You try a new diet, and so on. These measures may help in the short term, but the only long-term solution is to treat the syndrome itself: the imbalance of androgen hormone in your body.

Skin and hair problems cannot really be considered without an awareness of their psychological effects. Shining hair on the head and a clear, smooth, glowing skin serve no practical purpose, but appearance, especially that of women, is given a great deal of emphasis in our society. The skin and hair are the parts of the body that are most fully revealed to others. They are often the first things people notice. Deviance from what is considered socially acceptable in terms of appearance can make life difficult.

If you have hair on your face in places you don't want hair, or if your acne is persistent, people may shun you, think you have some infectious disease, or criticize you for lack of hygiene. Few would suspect that you are suffering from a hormone problem. Such is the taboo about excess hair in women that the problem is rarely discussed. Women have become so good at hiding it from others that even doctors fail to notice. As a result, those with the condition often think they are alone.

Should you have some of the symptoms of androgen disorder, it is highly likely that you have been blaming yourself rather than realizing you have a hormonal disorder that needs medical attention. You should not feel guilty about seeing a doctor. You are not vain; you just want to improve the quality of your life. If you spend an excessive amount of time removing unwanted hair or trying to conceal your acne, you should seek medical advice. You'll be helping not only yourself but also other sufferers. The more women come forward and bring androgen disorder to the attention of doctors, the more it will be perceived as a real health problem.

Facial hair and acne are common clinical conditions. They shouldn't be dismissed as merely cosmetic, because they are a source of emotional distress and as such deserve to be taken seriously. We can only hope that in time the medical profession will appreciate this and increase its understanding of the condition and how to manage it.

Those who have never suffered from serious skin and hair problems may not perceive them to be all that important. They fail to realize that these problems affect how we feel about ourselves. They can affect all areas of our lives, cause anxiety, and be a barrier to greater intimacy with others.

> When my acne finally cleared up, it was as if I had been living all my life with poor vision and then was given glasses. Everything felt better. I got my confidence back. Life seems brighter, clearer now.
>
> *Linda, age thirty-eight*

Facial and bodily hair will cause anxiety for many women. It is socially unacceptable. It is generally accepted in our society that men have hair on their face and body and women don't; therefore, having male hair growth must mean that a woman is too masculine. It is this kind of attitude that makes life so very hard for women with androgen disorder. Such an attitude, however, is based on ignorance and erroneous beliefs about the differences between the sexes.

Men and women are not quite as different as we would like to believe. "In fact, men and women have more similarities than differences," writes Dr. Geoffrey Redmond in *Women's Hormones* (p. 35). We share the same hormones, which control how our bodies function. Sufferers of androgen disorder are not "masculine" women. Characteristics that we imagine must belong to the opposite sex can actually be seen in us. Every woman has facial and bodily hair. Even celebrities and models have facial hair, but it is cleverly concealed by makeup and photography, creating an impossible ideal. If you have androgen disorder, you will simply have slightly more hair than is usual in a woman.

ANDROGEN DISORDER
AND THE ADRENAL GLAND

Changes in your appearance are most likely to occur if you have an adrenal gland disorder. This androgen disorder has been so neglected that there isn't really any medical term for it.

Adrenal gland disorder occurs when the increase in androgen production that occurs at puberty, *adrenarche*, is exaggerated and the gland starts to produce more androgen than is necessary. Or in some cases, the adrenal gland has gone through puberty normally and then suddenly starts to produce far higher amounts of testosterone than normal.

Redmond writes in *Women's Hormones* (p. 194) that androgen excess caused by adrenal gland problems is even more common than that caused by ovarian gland problems.

Why then does the latter receive all the attention? The answer is simple: ovarian gland problems are more likely to affect fertility. Fertility problems are always taken far more seriously by doctors than problems with how a woman looks and feels, which are the types of problems caused by adrenal gland disorders. These disorders can also cause menstrual abnormalities and infertility, but more often than not they will affect just appearance, which doctors tend to dismiss as a purely cosmetic concern. They may also cause chronic fatigue, which doctors often classify as a psychological problem.

What triggers this late onset or overproduction of androgens by the adrenal gland is as yet unknown. Doctors differ in their understanding of the causes. Some, like Dr. James Douglas, believe it is hereditary, while others think it is related to metabolic disturbances or stress, problems that directly affect the adrenal glands.

The adrenal glands control many body functions and play a crucial role in resistance to stress by releasing hormones to combat the stress. If you are constantly under stress, the adrenal glands reacts with an abnormal response. Androgen excess and the symptoms associated with it are likely to occur. In fact, Dr. Robert R. Franklin and Dorothy Kay Brochman, authors of *In Pursuit of Infertility* (p. 133), believe there is a strong connection between androgen disorder and stress. Other doctors, such as Redmond (*Women's Hormones*, p. 201), believe that stress is not the determining factor. The relationship between stress and androgen disorder will be discussed in more detail in chapter 4.

HIRSUTISM

> I have a mustache. My mother has one too. We both shave on a daily basis. I never go anywhere without my razor blade.
>
> *Rebecca, age forty*

Hirsutism is the medical term for an excess of facial and body hair in women. In these cases, hair grows in androgen-sensitive areas—that is, areas in which men are prone to grow hair, such as on the face, the midline of the chest around the nipples, and the lower back.

If you have hirsutism you are probably worried most about your appearance. You have to shave regularly. If you want to wear a bikini, you shave the hair on your lower abdomen and inner thighs. Maybe you have had the problem for so long you have just learned to live with it.

Hirsutism usually begins at puberty, but it can appear at any age. It can develop during pregnancy because of androgens from the placenta. It can also occur during and after menopause because of hormonal changes. Drugs such as dilantin, androgens, diaxoxide, and minoxidil can also cause hirsutism.

It is important to remember that not all women with androgen disorders have hirsutism, but about 90 percent do. Along with menstrual irregularity it is one of the most common symptoms. There are ethnic differences: Asian women, Nordic women, and Native American women rarely have this symptom. Mediterranean, Middle Eastern, and Caucasian women are the most likely to have the condition. Genetics also plays a part: the condition may be inherited. Also, some women can get hirsutism when there is no androgen disorder and the cause is unknown.

Idiopathic Hirsutism

Idiopathic hirsutism is the medical term used to describe the condition of a woman who has androgen levels that are normal but also has signs of androgen excess such as increased body hair. *Idiopathic* simply means that the cause is unknown, but many doctors believe that the problem is probably connected with excessive activity in the hair follicle due to an oversensitivity to androgens. Let me explain:

The critical amount of androgen hormone necessary for each woman will always be small, but it varies from woman to woman. Two women can have the same androgen level, and one will develop symptoms whereas another will not. Why does this happen?

It could be related to how tissues of the body react to androgen. Some women may have testosterone receptors that are more numerous or more sensitive than other women's. For instance, there will be normal levels of androgen but androgenic symptoms, like acne. The problem could still be said to be hormonal, although it is caused not by high levels of androgen but by how a woman's skin reacts to androgen.

Hair Follicles and Androgens

Hair follicles appear all over the body. However, the tendency to grow hair differs greatly in various parts of the body. We just don't grow hair on the palms of our hands, for example. This is because skin areas vary in how they respond to hormonal signals for hair growth. There are many kinds of hormonal signals and other factors involved, but androgens seem to have the greatest effect.

Androgens determine the type and distribution of hairs on your body.

Types of Hair

In general, there are three types of hair. *Lanugo* is the soft hair covering the fetus, which is shed in the early postpartum period. *Vellus* hairs are short (2–5mm), soft, and fine, and they cover the apparently hairless areas of the body. *Terminal* hairs are long and coarse, covering the scalp, pubic, and axillary (underarm) areas; the eyebrows and eyelashes are also made up of terminal hairs. Terminal hairs are transformed from the vellus hairs in sex-hormone-responsive hair follicles. The sensitivity of the transformation from vellus to terminal hair depends on genetic or racial background, the area of the body stimulated, and hormones that control hair growth.

Patterns of Hair Growth

There are three patterns of hair growth:

- Asexual hair growth, such as growth of the eyebrows and eyelashes and growth on the scalp.

- Ambisexual hair growth, such as terminal hairs in pubic and axillary areas stimulated in both men and women by androgens. If your androgen levels are normal, you will have ambisexual hair growth.

- Sexual hair growth, with male-pattern hair growth involving beard, chest hair, and so on. If your androgen levels are elevated, you will develop male hair-growth patterns here.

In the hair follicle, testosterone is converted to dihydrotestosterone (DHT). It is DHT that increases the thickness and coarseness of terminal hair and that stimulates the vellus-producing follicles to produce terminal hair. The effect of androgen on hair follicles depends on the area of the body where the hair grows. Some areas are resistant to androgen, but other areas are very sensitive. Ambisexual areas are sensitive to low levels of androgen. At puberty, when androgen levels rise, hair grows on the pubic area first. The next most androgen-sensitive area is the axillary or underarm area. The skin of the pubic and underarm areas also darkens in response to androgen stimulation and becomes more sensitive, which might have something to do with nature's way of drawing attention to the pubic area for the purposes of reproduction.

Cycles of Hair Growth

Unfortunately, even when androgen levels return to normal, the problems may not disappear immediately, because the life cycle of the hair will continue. This is because hair growth has three cycles: *anagen*, the phase of growth that is active and determines length; *catagen*, a transition stage; and *telogen*, when hair rests and then sheds. Depending on body location, hair follicles have totally different rhythms of activity. Hormonal treatment can be effective only during the last two stages of hair growth, so if the problem is chin and facial hair or scalp hair, which have a long anagen phase, it may take a year or so for treatment to be effective. This explains why male-pattern hirsutism can often be seen in women who have had elevated androgen levels in the past but whose androgen levels are now normal.

Alopecia

When I thought I was going bald when I was thirty-four, it was one of the most terrible moments of my life. I was filled with panic and fear.

Nancy, age forty-three

Alopecia is the medical term for hair loss. Female hair loss is seldom brought to our attention, even though about twenty million American women suffer from it. Being bald is perhaps even more socially unacceptable for a woman in our society than having acne or excess hair growth.

If you have always had a full head of hair, you may not understand how important hair is. But just think about our children's stories: the beautiful princess always has flowing locks and always gets her prince. Rapunzel even finds a prince by using her hair. A woman's hair is her crowning glory, the mark of her beauty, femininity, and desirability. A common punishment for women in centuries past was to shave their head, to cause them the ultimate in shame and humiliation. It is terribly unfair that men are allowed to go bald but women are not. A bald man can still be considered attractive to women, but a bald woman will generally not be viewed the same way.

There are many causes of alopecia, but one of them is linked to androgen disorder and is called *androgenic alopecia*. Basically what happens is that an excess of male hormone causes male-pattern baldness. Hair starts to thin at the back or crown of the head. Some women look like they have a high forehead because of their receding hairline.

Thinning hair that occurs with alopecia is not the same as the shedding of hair. We all lose hundreds of hairs each day, and normally new hair grows to replace the ones shed. However, if your hair is thinning as well, the normal shedding of hairs, which you will notice when you wash or brush your hair, can cause great alarm.

There are various degrees of hair loss. Mild cases may be noticeable to you but rarely to others. Only a little area of the scalp is visible. Then there are the more severe cases, in which more of the scalp is visible. Most women suffering from this problem manage to conceal it with clever hair dressing. Finally, there are the very severe cases in which the scalp is clearly visible. These are very rare and take a long time to develop.

Some women may not even notice their mild alopecia, but if you do notice some thinning, now is the time to seek treatment before it gets worse. It's not really advisable to hope that it will just get better without treatment, because there is no way of knowing how alopecia will develop if left untreated. Androgenic alopecia is unpredictable. It can appear gradually, but it can also appear suddenly. Finding a doctor who understands the condition and takes it seriously is not always easy.

You should not feel bad if losing your hair upsets you more than anything else in your life. "In my experience" writes Redmond in *Women's Hormones* (p. 261), "there are few physical changes as distressing to a woman as hair loss."

Nothing may devastate you more than hair loss. One of the first things cancer patients worry about when they start chemotherapy is the stigma of losing their hair. Our hair is an adornment; it expresses our individuality. Losing it is like losing a part of ourselves and how we express ourselves to the world. Whatever a woman's age, class, or race, going bald or losing hair is a miserable experience. If you suffer from severe alopecia, you will need counseling and support.

ACNE AND SKIN PROBLEMS

When I was twenty-five, I did go to see a doctor about my acne. The doctor told me that I should watch my diet, get some fresh air, and exercise and relax more. He also told me not to worry about my irregular periods, and heavy bleeding on some cycles, as lots of women have menstrual irregularity. He said I should only be concerned if I wanted to have a baby and suggested that I go on the Pill to regulate things. I resisted, preferring to use condoms for birth control.

At the time I was starting an exciting new job in advertising and putting a lot of pressure on myself to do well. Within two years I was promoted to a more senior position. I worked long hours and many weekends. There was always so much to do. It was around this time that my acne really began to flare up. I noticed how people looked at me when the condition was really bad. They probably thought I had a terrible diet, or didn't wash properly or something. It was awful, especially as in my career appearance does count. I am convinced that my acne was a problem for some of my managers. I also got scarring from old spots. I tried creams, lotions, face packs, herbal remedies, changes in diet. Nothing seemed to work.

My boyfriend never complained, but sometimes when my face was bad I just did not want to get intimate. When my periods stopped for five months I was scared I might be pregnant. Home tests read negative, but I went to my doctor to make sure. The doctor suspected that I had a hormonal disorder and that this was causing my acne and irregular periods. He said that going on the Pill, something I never wanted to do, would help both problems at the same time.

I'm on the Pill now. It makes me feel sick and heavy in the mornings, but thank goodness my acne has finally cleared up after all those years. Its also a huge relief to have regular, painless periods.

Rebecca, age thirty-seven

Recent studies show that up to 50 percent of adults between the ages of twenty and forty have some form of acne. One in nine adults will consult a doctor about acne every year.

Acne and skin problems during the massive hormonal shifts of puberty are quite usual. Everyone gets oilier skin at puberty. Some will get acne, but the problem is usually mild and it goes away. We all get the occasional spot or pimple, especially just before a period, and this is nothing to worry about. If, however, acne is persistent in your twenties and beyond, there is cause for concern.

Dr. Tony Chu, an honorary consultant dermatologist at Hammersmith Hospital in London and founder of the Acne

Support Group (see Resources section), thinks that the reason adults suffer from acne is a "switch mechanism that usually turns on at puberty and switches off after about five years. But in some people, especially women, the switch is delayed and turns on later, perhaps triggered by stress or having a baby. The switch always turns back off again, but there is no way of predicting when that will happen" (*The Sunday Times, Style*, January 9, 1998, p. 27).

Nobody knows for sure what causes adult acne, but most doctors agree that there is a strong hormonal connection. Why else would we be more prone to it during times of hormonal change, such as puberty or pregnancy? Even though the connection seems obvious, millions of women don't see a doctor about the problem and instead blame themselves for poor hygiene or diet.

Excess androgen may cause the problem (Redmond, *Women's Hormones*, p. 173), or it could be triggered by an abnormal reaction of the skin to normal levels of testosterone. It is not caused by chocolate, fatty food, cakes, and sweets, although sometimes they can make the condition worse. Poor hygiene will aggravate the problem, but it is not the cause either.

The excess androgen that causes acne is probably produced as a reaction to stress, which makes the adrenal glands overproduce stress hormones and androgen. *Executive acne* is a term that has arisen to explain why both men and women suffer from it as they climb the corporate ladder. Androgens act on the sebaceous glands to increase the production of sebum (an oily protective secretion), which has to escape to the surface of the skin. When there is too much androgen, too much sebum is produced. Often the skin surface protein *keratin* becomes too sticky and prevents fluid from coming out of the sebaceous gland, by sealing it off. Bacteria then starts to grow. The oil increases pressure against the spot where it is sealed off, and it may break and form swelling. The cysts that occur with acne are almost like boils. When they finally break off, they can cause scarring of the skin and redness. Sometimes the spots can be so large that they hurt.

Women with high androgen levels have more sebum and are more at risk of acne, but not all will get acne. In addition, there are other factors that contribute to the development of acne, such as bacteria growing on the skin surface or an overactive immune system. Facial skin is most sensitive to the oil-stimulating effects of androgens. Acne can and does occur on other androgen-sensitive areas, such as the chest and back, but this is not usually the case. It is one of life's cruelties that acne most often affects the face and not an area of the body that you can easily conceal.

COMPLEXION

My face just seems to look pale and tired all the time.
Amanda, age twenty-eight

Age-dependent skin changes may be influenced by androgen disorders, because aging of the skin is linked to our hormones. Too much sebum production can affect your complexion. Healthy skin should have a shine and glow. We spend much of our lives trying to enhance or capture that healthy, shining look with cosmetics and makeup. A dull complexion usually goes hand-in-hand with acne, but sometimes there is no acne but just a dull complexion.

Dull skin can be caused by many factors, such as lack of sunlight, poor eating habits, and lack of sleep. But when the skin constantly looks unhealthy, a hormonal imbalance is likely to be the cause.

It seems logical that a dull complexion could be the result of an imbalance of the sex hormones, but this connection is rarely made by medical researchers. Women spend millions of dollars each year on soaps, cleansers, and cosmetics to improve the condition of their skin. However, if there is an androgen excess, no amount of washing and cleansing will make the problem go away. It is androgenic hormones that keep the sebaceous glands secreting oil and give the complexion that oily, gray look.

If your skin has the correct amount of estrogen and androgen, you will look radiant. If you have excess androgen, your skin will probably look pasty and colorless You just look better if there is not too much androgen circulating.

UNDERARM ODOR

My aerobics teacher told me about my body odor problem. One day after class she suggested I watch my personal hygiene, as other class members were complaining. She probably felt as embarrassed as I about it. I felt terrible and never went back to her class again.

Sarah, age twenty-five

During puberty, increased levels of androgen produce body odor in both boys and girls. Developing body odor in the underarms is normal in both men and women. An extra dose of it at puberty is not unusual and is not always due to poor hygiene. The odor is produced by an increase in androgen levels. Regular washing will help, but not until the hormonal shifts of puberty have passed will body odor decrease.

An excessive amount of body odor after puberty may be caused by excess androgen. Many women with this problem manage to hide it as best they can with zealous washing and deodorants. Others, however, are not aware that they have a problem. They tend to be shunned, or worse still, unfairly ridiculed and criticized. While body odor is normal, if you are spending large amounts of time trying to control what seems to be excessive body odor, you may wish to check out the possibility of androgen overproduction.

VIRILIZATION OR MASCULINIZATION

Women with virilization or masculinization start to lose scalp hair. Their breasts shrink, and they develop severe hirsutism. There could be an increase in muscle mass, as well as weight gain in the upper part of the body. Basically the body becomes more masculine and loses its femininity. Sometimes the voice deepens so much that women find it hard to sing the high notes they used to.

Most women with androgen disorder have androgen levels that are higher than normal, but nowhere near the same level as men have in their bodies. For virilization to occur, androgen levels need to be massive, and the chances of this happening are very low. When virilization does occur, it is usually sudden and associated with some kind of serious disease, like a tumor, or the use of steroids.

Tumors

Masculinization is associated with adrenal and ovarian tumors, which are rare conditions. It can be accompanied by pain and weight loss.

Adrenal tumors are very dangerous but also very rare. Diagnosis is established by a scan of the adrenal, and the tumors tend to be large. Ovarian tumors are more common. Again, they can be detected by scanning. They are generally smaller and usually not malignant.

DISORDERS OF SEXUAL DIFFERENTIATION

Androgens play a crucial role in sexual differentiation of the fetus at the level of internal and external genitalia. If these hormones are absent, or not working properly, fetal development is affected and disorders of sexual differentiation may occur.

Guevedore syndrome is a perplexing condition. Children born as girls turn into boys at puberty. About twenty-five years ago, the condition was discovered in the village of Salinas in the Dominican Republic by Julianne Imperato-McGinley and her research team. The individuals concerned were referred to by the villagers as *guevedoce* (penis at age twelve) or *machihembra* (first woman then man).

McGinley proposed that conditions like guevedore syndrome are the direct result of some form of antagonism to androgen. For some reason, in these people testosterone does not work properly.

There are also babies who are born female and have ovaries but who have ambiguous-looking genitals or some other confusion between maleness and femaleness. This is not full-blown hermaphrodism, an extremely rare condition when both ovaries and testes are present, but the more common form of *pseudo-hermaphrodism.* The problem here may again be related to androgen. Many doctors believe that the condition is triggered by exposure of the fetus to an excess of androgen in the womb before the fetus is twelve weeks old. After twelve weeks, androgens will only cause an enlargement of the clitoris and not other abnormalities. Before twelve weeks, though, excess androgens can lead to masculinization of the external genitalia. The exposure of female fetuses to androgens (through high androgen levels in the mother's blood) is very unusual. When it does happen, these children can be treated to prevent further excess androgen production.

Plastic surgery will repair the external genitalia, but there are alternatives to surgery. The Intersex Society of North America is one of many activist groups calling for no longer seeing intersexed genitals as abnormal. Their Web site is at www.isna.org.

PRECOCIOUS AND DELAYED PUBERTY

Rebecca was a beautiful baby. She weighed nearly nine pounds at birth and was perfectly healthy. Apart from the usual baby traumas, she was easy to deal with. She made her parents very proud and happy. Her growth was normal up until age six, when she suddenly had an unusual growth spurt. Tiny hairs began to grow on her pubic and underarm areas. Her mother was concerned, but she did not really worry until she began to notice an unpleasant body odor that persisted even though she bathed Rebecca daily. A few months passed and Rebecca's mother began to get anxious. The pubic and underarm hair were getting thicker. She wondered what was happening to her daughter. A month or so later, she realized that her little girl was developing small breasts, and this had nothing to do with weight gain. She did not take her daughter to the doctor, though, until Rebecca was in the bathroom one day and screamed, "Mommy, I'm bleeding!"

Rebecca had started her periods before her seventh birthday.

Mom and Dad were assured by the doctor, after he had run a series of tests, that Rebecca did not have some deadly disease. What was abnormal was that she was entering puberty at an usually young age. Testosterone production had started prematurely, causing pubic hair growth and body odor. Androgen production had later been followed by early production of estrogen. These hormones had triggered Rebecca's adult development. She was placed on hormonal treatment, which stopped the breast growth and menstruation, but she still kept growing at a faster rate than her contemporaries.

Apart from becoming at little more demanding and irritable, Rebecca was not affected by the whole experience. It was not easy for her parents, though. Mom was afraid that Rebecca's premature physical development would mean that she would experience a premature sex drive. She became extremely protective of her daughter and limited her contact with boys. Although she never noticed an increase in flirting with boys, she was not prepared for the uncomfortable feelings the problem aroused in her. She mourned the loss of her daughter's childhood innocence. She found it hard to bond with her daughter. This child-woman sometimes seemed like a stranger. How was she supposed to treat her: as the child she was or the young adult she appeared to be? Dad also had some anxious moments. He was terrified that his daughter would be taken advantage of at too young an age. His little girl had breasts, hips, and pubic hair, but psychologically and mentally she was still a child.

When Rebecca, now twenty-two, sees photographs of herself at age seven she feels that somehow she missed out on her childhood. She cannot remember a time when she did not have to wear bras, shave under her arms, and use deodorant and tampons. There is a sense of loss. She worries that when she has children the same will happen to them.

When a child goes through puberty he or she will transform into a man or a woman. We have all been through it. We all know what it involves and what to expect and that it can be a time of conflict and confusion for adolescents and their families. Just imagine how traumatic it must be if puberty is premature. Equally traumatic is a delayed puberty.

I never felt like I belonged anywhere. I never really had any friends. My birthdays were sad and lonely. I had no boyfriend during my teens. The kids at school thought I was weird. I had no interest in sex at all, boys or girls. I hated my body. I tried everything I could to cover it up. Gym classes were a nightmare. Everyone would tease me when I was in the shower.

Why?

Because my bones stuck out. You could probably have counted the number of vertebrae on my back. I didn't need a bra. I had no breasts. I had no pubic hair at all.

There were nights when I lay in bed crying. I longed to be like everyone else, but I wasn't. The doctors who examined me said that I was suffering from hormonal imbalance. I just didn't have enough androgen and estrogen to help me grow up.

Kristin, age twenty

There are many theories circulating about what triggers puberty. One of the most convincing is the theory that a certain body weight must be reached before it occurs. We also know, however, that puberty is connected with the action of both androgens and estrogens.

Although the onset of puberty may occur as early as age five or six, and there are even reports of girls becoming pregnant at six, sexual development under the age of eight is described as *precocious puberty*. The adrenal gland, which produces androgen, and the ovarian gland, which produces estrogen, become active at a much earlier age due to stimulation by the pituitary gland.

True precocity is when a girl develops early because of the premature release of hormonal signals to initiate puberty. Pituitary signals simply start too early. In most cases this happens for no apparent reason and a child will have an excess amount of androgen and estrogen circulating in the blood. Breast enlargement, underarm hair, pubic hair, and menstrual bleeding will develop. Bones develop rapidly and then stop growing prematurely, leaving the girl with short stature. Often in cases of androgen excess, the voice deepens and there is enlargement of the clitoris.

False precocity is the name given to sexual development that occurs without the ovaries maturing at the same time. This is the truest form of androgen disorder at puberty. There is an excess of androgen causing underarm and pubic hair, body odor, and muscle buildup without breast development and menstrual bleeding. It can be caused by defects in the adrenal glands or an adrenal or ovarian gland tumor.

When the adrenals start to produce androgenss, the event is called *adrenarche*. When it occurs too early, it is called *precocious adrenarche*. It is not necessarily harmful, but it can be distressing. For instance, many misconceive the body odor to be the result of a lack of cleanliness. This is not the case. The odor is produced by the action of androgens on sweat and resulting changes in the normal bacteria.

Precocious sexual maturation is five times more common in girls than in boys. In 10 percent of cases it runs in families. It can be caused by an underlying disorder, like an infection in the hypothalamus, such as meningitis, or a tumor in or near the hypothalamus, the small area at the base of the brain that controls most basic bodily functions. These tumors are usually not malignant, but they can cause damage by pressing on other vital structures. Some of these tumors never grow, but others do and might need to be surgically removed. Whenever puberty starts early, tumors in the ovaries must also be considered. That is why precocious puberty should always be monitored carefully when it occurs.

When sexual development occurs after the age of fourteen in girls, it is called *delayed puberty*. In girls there will be a failure to develop breasts, lack of menstruation, and absence of pubic and body hair. For some reason the body is unable to produce the sex hormones estrogen and androgen, which are responsible for these changes. This condition is called *hypogonadotropic hypogonadism* (HH), and it occurs when there is not enough brain hormone (the gonadotropins FSH and LH) to stimulate the adrenals and ovaries. Sometimes this condition is permanent, but most often it is not, and the pituitary will eventually produce the hormones that initiate puberty. But it can result in physical abnormalities, such as widely spaced nipples or defects in the cardiovascular system. Genetic factors may delay the secretion of sex hormones. Stress and malnutrition are also contributory factors, as are chronic diseases, brain defects, and tumors in the endocrine glands.

Both precocious and premature puberty are potentially dangerous conditions. If you think you child is developing too quickly or too slowly for his or her age, go to see your doctor. In almost all cases, hormonal therapy can rectify the problem.

ANDROGEN IMBALANCES
CAUSED BY BRAIN DEFECTS

Sometimes rare androgen-related disorders, such as precocious puberty or gender identity problems, are caused by brain defects or tumors that affect the hypothalamus or the pituitary. The hypothalamus or pituitary are unable to stimulate the adrenal or ovarian glands, and confusing signals are sent to the glands. A tumor can interfere with the normal feedback system that keeps the hormones in balance.

Androgen imbalances such as Cushing's disease (see below), hermaphrodism, and precocious and delayed puberty can all be caused by brain injuries or disorders, such as inflammation of the brain, a brain abscess, infections, head injuries, tumors, and brain cysts. The proper functioning of the brain can also be affected by X-rays of the head, infections, syphilis, and injury to the head.

When androgen imbalance is due to brain disorders, the imbalance can be severe and very dangerous. It must be stressed, however, that these conditions are extremely rare indeed. They have simply been included here to show you the incredible range of androgen disorder and how it can range from the mild, but still distressing, effects it can have on your skin and hair to the devastating effects of severe masculinization.

CUSHING'S DISEASE

Cushing's disease occurs when certain hormones, including androgen, cortisol, estrogen, and aldosterone, are overproduced by the adrenal gland. The disease is most common in women, especially young and middle-aged women. It can be caused by an overdose of corticosteroids, taken for a variety of reasons, such as for arthritis, Crown's disease, bodybuilding, or tumors in the pituitary gland or adrenal gland itself or in other parts of the body.

People with Cushing's syndrome have a distinctive appearance: large stomach, rounded back, fat face and neck, and thin arms and legs due to muscle wastage. Other symptoms include thin and dry skin, a tendency to bruise easily, discoloration of the skin, hairiness, puffy eyes, backache, mood swings, acne, hirsutism, diabetes, high blood pressure, infertility, and growth retardation.

USE OF STEROIDS

While most of this chapter has been devoted to the signs and symptoms of androgen disorder, a word is needed here about one other common factor that causes symptoms of androgen disorder. This is the use of steroids, which are usually taken to affect a person's appearance.

> I love to see how people gasp when they see me. They don't expect to see such strength in a woman. I worked hard to look this way. Sure, I've taken the odd steroid or two to give me a boost. Why do I do that? Because I am addicted to looking this way. I could not go back to looking thin and weak.
>
> *Lucy, age thirty*

When I started out in bodybuilding I was ambitious. I wanted to be the best. I worked hard to build up my muscles, was disciplined about my diet, and had a positive attitude. But I was not winning competitions, and I wanted to. A friend of mine suggested I try a few steroids. It was amazing. After just a few months my muscle definition improved so much that I came in fourth in a regional competition. The following year I came in first. The fact that the high level of testosterone I was pumping into my body gave me facial hair, acne, irregular periods, and a deeper voice seemed a small price to pay at the time.

Looking back, I think I must have been crazy to abuse my body like that.

Margaret, age thirty-four

Androgen disorders that change your appearance can be caused by ingestion of anabolic steroids and certain medications, such as cyclosporine, danazol, phenytoin, glucocorticoids, minoxidil, and dioxide. Certain anabolic drugs, such as dilantin, also cause an increase in muscle mass and hair growth.

Since testosterone has a tissue-building or anabolic effect, steroids are prescribed by doctors for certain diseases. Steroids can be very helpful drugs when used for medicinal purposes. For example, the starving victims of the Nazi war camps were treated with steroids to get their strength and body weight back to normal. Testosterone is also used to treat certain blood diseases, such as anemia and kidney- and muscle-wasting cancers.

It is the nonmedical use of steroids that causes concern. Both male and female athletes use them to enhance muscle size and strength. Bodybuilding is probably the most prominent women's sport in which the use of steroids is prevalent. However, statistics show that women marathon runners, track and field athletes, and tennis players also use them. The major effects of the anabolic steroids on the female athlete are an increase in blood volume, a probable increase in skeletal muscle size and strength, an enhancement of endurance, a reduction in percentage of body fat, increased muscle mass, changes in distribution of body fat, and alterations in the menstrual cycle.

It is not only athletes who use steroids. Because steroids increase calorie-burning muscle power, some women take them in the misguided belief that the steroids will help them lose weight and tone their bodies, the desire for slenderness being the overriding concern.

Nonmedical use of steroids can cause troublesome side effects. If you are taking steroids to change the way you look, you are at risk of androgen disorder. Some women will experience a deepening of the voice, growth of facial hair, coarsening of the skin, hair loss, and cessation of menses. Some of these changes can become permanent, and the risk increases with higher doses. The herbs sarsaparilla and saw palmetto can be used to help boost testosterone levels and athletic performance naturally.

We will now turn our attention to perhaps the most common symptom of androgen disorder: menstrual irregularity.

4

Menstrual Abnormality and Infertility

I haven't had a period in six months now. I'm not pregnant. What's going on?

Nancy, age twenty-six

My periods have always been irregular, but in the last year or so they have become wildly unpredictable. I'll go for months without a period and then I'll have a long, heavy bleed. Should I see a doctor?

Robin, age thirty-two

The most common medical effect of androgen disorder is menstrual irregularity. In fact, androgen imbalance is the leading cause of menstrual dysfunction.

The medical terms for menstrual dysfunction prior to menopause are *amenorrhea* and *oligomenorrhea*. Oligomenorrhea refers to having only the occasional period. Amenorrhea refers to the total absence of menstrual function. Primary amenorrhea refers to having never had a period. Secondary amenorrhea refers to cycles that once occurred but that have now stopped.

Contrary to popular belief, menstrual irregularity is not perfectly normal and "just one of those things." If your periods are constantly irregular, there is something wrong.

The normal menstrual cycle lasts around twenty-eight days from the first day of bleeding in one cycle to the first day of bleeding in the next. Periods—the time when bleeding occurs—last about five days within that cycle. Periods are rarely that exact and will vary within six or seven days. Basically, a normal time between periods is twenty-one to thirty-five days. Occasionally you will have cycles that are even shorter or longer than this, and that is nothing to worry about, but if your cycles are repeatedly shorter or longer you should get medical attention. Every woman's menstrual cycle is unique to her, and sometimes extreme regularity will not indicate a hormonal problem, but more often than not it does.

Many doctors underestimate how significant a normal menstrual cycle is for a woman's health and well-being emotionally, mentally, and physically. For many years scant attention has been paid to the menstrual cycle, unless fertility is an issue. The attitude has been that having a period is significant only if you are trying to get pregnant. Time and time again women have gone to doctors with menstrual problems and been told that there is nothing to worry about.

Thankfully, doctors are now realizing what women have always intuitively sensed: missed periods and other kinds of menstrual irregularity are significant. Think about your own cycle: when you are irregular, you just don't feel right. We may not know all that much about how our bodies work, but we do know that we are supposed to have a monthly bleed from puberty to menopause. This is how our bodies are designed. A regular cycle is an indicator of good health and reassures us of our potential for fertility.

A healthy menstrual cycle is the best indicator we have of our general good health. When a woman's body is healthy, she will menstruate regularly. When her health is poor, the menstrual cycle usually starts to show signs of irregularity. For instance, amenorrhea will occur during times of disease and illness. In response to the stress placed on the body, the reproductive cycle switches off to conserve energy needed for healing. During illness there is a big energy drain on the body, and many women may experience absent or infrequent menses. Even a heavy cold can cause a disruption in the menstrual routine. Usually periods return when full health is recovered. In cases of serious illness, however, such as kidney or liver failure, cystic fibrosis, diabetes, or pituitary or ovarian tumors, amenorrhea may be long-term or become permanent.

We can tolerate only so much stress in a given period of time. When the body is trying to cope under stress, it needs all the energy it can get. Stress can affect the hormonal feedback of the hypothalamus, pituitary, and ovarian glands, which govern the menstrual cycle. The reproductive cycle is not vital to sustain your life, so your body will prioritize when energy levels are dangerously low and sacrifice menstruation to conserve energy.

"You can't fool the body," says Sarah Berga, Ph.D., associate professor of obstetrics, gynecology, and psychiatry at the University of Pittsburgh. "Your body knows. It makes a judgment call. It knows that it is being mistreated, and since it won't have enough energy to maintain vital functioning, it gets 'rid' of the reproductive cycle. And no doctor can tell a patient exactly when it will turn back on again" (quoted in Anne Hogg, "Breaking the Cycle"). So, if you have been skipping periods on a regular basis, it is important that you go to see a doctor. Missed periods are a warning sign no woman should ignore.

ESTROGEN LEVELS

If problems occur in the first half of the reproductive cycle, before ovulation, menstruation will stop because there is not enough estrogen to prepare for menstruation.

Estrogen deficiency affects how you feel. Mood swings are common, and you may have hot flashes. There may be problems with your circulatory system. Estrogen-deficient women are at increased risk of heart disease and osteoporosis. You may also notice a reduction in breast size, poor vision, tooth and hair loss, vaginal dryness, and frequent urination.

Most women with androgen disorders are not necessarily estrogen-deficient. In some cases there may be an abundance of estrogen. This is because androgen disorders typically affect the second half of the cycle. Estrogen levels rise as usual, but for some reason no egg is released, and so even more estrogen will be produced, leading to a condition referred to as *estrogen dominance*.

In his important study "What Your Doctor May Not Tell You About Menopause," Dr. John R. Lee explains clearly the many effects estrogen and progesterone have on women and the characteristics of estrogen dominance. These include bloating, irregular periods, weight gain around the hips and thighs, sugar cravings, fatigue, and diminished sex drive.

Symptoms of androgen disorder show up when androgen levels rise above or fall below the level that is right for you, regardless of what is happening with your other hormones. If you have problems with your estrogen and progesterone levels, this does not mean you will have problems with your androgen levels too. But androgen imbalance is more likely to occur when other hormones, such as estrogen, are out of balance, because the hormonal system is so interconnected.

ANOVULATION

Women with high androgen levels tend to have *anovulatory* menstrual cycles, which means that they do not ovulate. No egg is ever released from the ovary. Normal ovulation usually takes place around day fourteen of a menstrual cycle, leaving around ten days for an egg to be fertilized, if pregnancy were to occur. If you have at least eight or nine periods a year you are probably ovulating, but if your periods are irregular you need to find out whether you are ovulating. You can do this by getting any of the home ovulation kits available in drugstores. You can also check for a temperature increase around the time of ovulation or for your vaginal discharge to be clear and sticky, like egg whites.

How anovulation affects each woman will vary. Some will stop menstruating altogether, others will still have infrequent bleeding, others will have heavy periods that are longer than usual. All will be temporarily infertile. The higher the levels of estrogen, the thicker the buildup of endometrium (the lining of the uterus)and the heavier the period. Progesterone released after ovulation in a normal cycle limits the amount of bleeding that occurs by contracting the blood vessels in the uterus. Without progesterone, a woman is likely to experience heavy bleeding (hypermenorrhea), periods that last too long (menorrhagia), periods that are too frequent (polymenorrhea), bleeding that is too frequent as well as too long (menometrorrhagia), or bleeding between cycles (breakthrough bleeding).

Women with androgen disorders are usually anovulatory and develop a complex disorder known as polycystic ovary syndrome.

POLYCYSTIC OVARY SYNDROME

In my opinion, the most common androgen disorder is some-thing called polycystic ovary syndrome. It accounts for around 80 to 90 percent of the androgen disorders we see in women.

Dr. James Douglas

When excessive androgens inhibit follicular development and cysts develop in the ovaries to produce even more androgen, this condition is called *polycystic ovary syndrome* (PCOS). PCOS is the most usual cause of menstrual irregularity.

PCOS is an extremely complicated disorder in which excess androgen from the adrenals and ovaries causes the brain to send confusing signals to the ovaries. Often, high levels of estrogen throw the hormonal ratio out of balance. Follicles start to mature but fail to ripen properly. The outer lining of the ovary becomes thicker, making it hard for the eggs to break out. Without a hormonal trigger, eggs are never released and follicles continue to make hormones. When follicles fail to mature they stay in the ovaries and make more androgen hormone so that even more is circulating in the body. Over time, more and more trapped follicles build up in the ovaries so that they become filled with cysts and hard fibrotic growth. The outer lining of the ovary becomes thick and inhibits ovulation. Without ovulation, normal menstrual function cannot occur. The most sensitive test for PCOS is a transvaginal ultrasound. The characteristic appearance of PCOS is a ring of small to medium follicles around the circumference of an enlarged ovary.

Usually this condition begins just after puberty, but it takes time to develop and the polycystic appearance of the ovaries may not be detected until the twenties or thirties, when the symptoms become more severe. Prior to that, symptoms probably manifest in a mild way but are ignored and dismissed because they seem so mild—the odd missed period, for instance, or bout of acne past puberty. Weight gain, hirsutism, acne, irregular periods, infertility, and increased risk of cancer of the lining of the uterus are associated with PCOS. Masculinization sometimes occurs, but this is not usual.

Some women can have this condition without experiencing any of the symptoms except disturbances in ovulation. In mild cases, ovulation may just be a little more infrequent than usual, and there may or may not be problems with fertility. When this is the case the condition is called PCO—polycystic ovary—and not PCOS—polycystic ovary syndrome.

If there is high androgen and menstrual irregularity, a woman is usually considered to have PCO even if the ovary does not appear to have its characteristic cysts. The condition is diagnosed according to how the ovary functions, not how it appears.

The term *polycystic ovary* was coined by Dr. Nancy L. Stein and Dr. Bennett Leventhal in 1935. They noticed that some of their patients had irregular periods, obesity, excess body hair, and ovaries enlarged by cysts. Medical researchers now think that the condition may not have anything to do with cysts. Cysts are not always a factor. An interesting discussion appears in *Reproductive Endocrinology,* edited by Dr. S. C. Yen and Dr. Robert B. Jaffe. Yen argues that the condition begins at puberty and is associated with elevated androgen production from the adrenals and ovaries.

The condition is still poorly understood, but the label PCO has stuck. So if you are diagnosed with PCO, don't let the word *cyst* alarm you. Remember that *cyst* is an unfortunate name for what is just an unusual appearance of the ovaries caused by androgen excess, which can be effectively treated. Tumors are associated with PCO but are very rare. If you have too much male hormone you should not assume that, because it is unnatural and should not be there, cancer is inevitable.

Possible Causes of PCO and PCOS

Recent research indicates that certain types of hormonal disorder may be inherited. A genetic predisposition leads to the ovaries producing too much androgen. Daughters of patients with PCO do seem at a higher risk of getting the disease, but so far there have been no careful, systematic, conclusive studies.

According to Douglas, "a familial disposition to the condition is not uncommon. In other words if mothers have irregular periods, because their androgens are too high, their daughters usually have irregular periods for the same reason. That may or may not be a direct genetic link, but if your mother has it, you are much more likely to have it too."

PROBLEMS IN THE HORMONAL FEEDBACK LOOP

Women with androgen disorder have a slight abnormality in the endocrine feedback loop involving the hypothalamus, pituitary, ovaries, and adrenals. Somewhere along the line things get confused.

According to Douglas, "We don't often know where there is an abnormality. In cases of polycystic ovary, for instance, is this an abnormality with the hypothalamus, pituitary, or ovary? Is the defect in the brain or ovary? We don't have any idea yet. The hypothalamus and the pituitary send signals that stimulate the ovary. The ovary then sends back its chemical signals. It's a cycle. When you have something that's a cycle, where does the cycle start?"

Problems with the hormonal feedback loop may involve one or all of the glands. For instance, the hypothalamus sends out a signal to the pituitary. The pituitary malfunctions and as a result, too much androgen is created by the ovaries and the adrenals. Or the hypothalamus, pituitary, and adrenals do their job properly, but there are problems with the ovary and it overproduces androgen. Why this happens is still a great mystery. It is conceivable that some women are born with a genetic predisposition to problems with hormones. Some doctors also think that obesity and insulin levels, discussed in the next chapter, play a part. Others believe that stress is an important factor.

STRESS

Like many women who have PCO, Rebecca looked tired and anxious. She has been living with stress for many, many years.

"I just can't believe that he walked out on me," says Nancy, age fifty-one, wiping her eyes. "We have been together twenty-four years. What hurts even more is that he is getting on with his life, but its been a year now and I still can't get over the divorce. I spend most of my time crying."

"I live alone. I miss my mum and dad; they died years ago and my only sister lives in London. I never had children. It's probably too late now. I feel very lonely sometimes," says Belinda, age thirty-eight.

All these women have some form of PCO.

The idea that stress is a major cause of illness is popular, but the relationship between stress and PCOS is still a matter of debate in medical circles. Dr. Geoffrey Redmond (*Women's Hormones*, p. 201) believes that although the condition itself causes stress, there is no evidence that stress causes it. He adds that the theory that the condition is caused by stress encourages self-blame, which makes matters worse. Dr. Douglas believes that androgen disorders tend to be hereditary. If a woman is genetically predisposed to the disorder, however healthy her lifestyle, she will suffer from the disorder.

On the other hand, there are doctors who believe that there is some kind of connection between high levels of stress and problems with the endocrine system.

According to Dr. Robert R. Franklin and Dorothy Kay Brockman (*In Pursuit of Fertility*, p. 132), "When you have too much stress in your life—especially if this occurs in the teens when the ovaries are beginning to cycle—your chances of developing menstrual irregularity later in life significantly increase . . . excessive stress causes the adrenal glands to increase androgen production . . . the problem may start as early as the womb. If a pregnant woman has too much stress it will affect her unborn baby's hypothalamus so that it will not cycle properly at puberty."

Franklin and Brockman argue that stress overstimulates the adrenal glands, and if this happens repeatedly they become over-active and secrete too much androgen. The adrenal glands are our body's shock absorbers. The hormones they produce help us respond to stress as well as maintain energy and emotional bal-ance. When the body recognizes stress, the brain alerts the adrenal glands. In response, the adrenal glands secrete stress hor-mones and androgen. The excess androgen inhibits ovulation. Lack of ovulation causes the ovaries to secrete even more testos-terone. Over time, many or all of the symptoms of full-blown PCOS will develop, such as irregular periods, infertility, weight gain, acne, excessive hair growth, diabetes, or high blood pres-sure. Anxiety and depression are likely too.

Stress can be caused by major life changes, such as divorce or the death of a loved one, but even changes in routine, eating habits, travel arrangements, or place of residence will challenge the body as it tries to adapt to the new way of doing things. Sometimes even activities considered pleasurable, such as wed-dings or holidays, can be stressful. Our thoughts, feelings, and moods can also be stressful.

It is now believed that people who live alone release more cortisol into their bloodstream. Increased levels of cortisol are associated with androgen disorder. Cortisol also impairs the immune system, raises blood pressure, and elevates heart rate.

Dr. Dean Ornish, in *Love and Survival: The Scientific Basis for the Healing Power of Intimacy*, argues that our very survival depends on the healing power of love, intimacy, and relationships. According to Ornish, the real problem in the modern world is what he calls "emotional and spiritual heart disease." By this he means the lone-liness, isolation, and depression that have become so common today since the weakening of the community and family unit.

Ornish suggests that love and intimacy are the most powerful and meaningful interventions in a person's life, and that without them illness is more likely. Physicians too often concentrate on the physical and mechanistic—drugs, surgery, genes, and so on—ignoring the importance of love. Love and intimacy, for Dr. Ornish, are what can make us healthy and help us relax.

Physical stresses as well as emotional ones can affect the secretion of adrenal androgen. Infection, fever, exposure to hot and cold, increased physical activity, certain drugs, or addictions to smoking, alcohol, or drugs will stress your body. Not only will your health be poor due to a weakened immune system, but you are more likely to have some kind of hormonal imbalance.

Certain professions, such as medicine, fire fighting, or operating dangerous machinery, can be stressful if we can't build up the stamina to deal with them. Flight attendants also perform a highly stressful job. They must deal with a demanding public, and their adrenal glands are constantly forced to react to noise pollution, high altitudes, and changes in light cycle. It has been proved on animals that stress of this sort stops ovulation: if a rat is exposed to bright lights or loud noises over time, it will cease ovulating. Another place where we are seeing more and more instances of stress-induced menstrual irregularity and androgen imbalance is the world of female sport.

OVEREXERCISE

I love running and working out. It's my life. I teach exercise and aerobics and weight training. I also compete in marathons. I guess I'm lucky. I have always had a strong, muscular body and exercise comes easy to me. I've never had a problem with stamina and endurance. Some days I work out four or five hours, as well as teaching and training others.

I think I'm very fit and healthy. I just don't have any periods, though. My doctor tells me this is because my body is producing too many male hormones. I am afraid to seek treatment. I don't want to lose all the strength and stamina I have worked so hard to achieve. Suppressing my androgen level might make that happen. Not having periods feels wrong, but I'll worry about it if I decide to have a baby.

Mandy, age thirty-three

It is now common for women to be active participants in competitive and recreational physical activity. There is still great uncertainty, though, regarding how much intense physical activity can affect the hormonal balance of our bodies. As more of us participate in exercise and sport, and training programs become more strenuous, physicians are seeing an increase in complaints of menstrual cycle disturbances.

As early as the first century, Soranus of Ephesus mentioned in his treatise *On the Diseases of Women* that "amenorrhea is frequently observed in the youthful, the aged, the pregnant, in singers and those who take too much exercise." Recent studies prove that if intense training is begun before puberty, menarche (a girl's first period) is delayed, and if it begins after menarche, periods may stop.

Menstrual dysfunction, a classic symptom of androgen disorder, is a problem that affects many female athletes, especially those involved in high-intensity and weight-conscious sports. Researchers Hetland, Haarbo, Christiansen, and Larsen examined the menstrual cycle of two hundred runners and found that elite runners, who ran up to eighty miles a week, were at the greatest risk of developing amenorrhea.

Whereas approximately 5 percent of American women have three or fewer periods a year, in female athletes this percentage rises to 50 percent. A 1997 study by Johnson and Whitaker showed that amenorrhea affected 50 percent of competitive runners, 44 percent of ballet dancers, 25 percent of noncompetitive runners, and 12 percent of cyclists, gymnasts, and swimmers.

Low to moderate exercise—say, running fifteen to twenty miles a week—does not seem to alter the cycle greatly, but anything more than this becomes borderline and will more than likely result in menstrual abnormalities. Even recreational joggers demonstrate poor follicular development, hormonal imbalance, and absent ovulation.

More and more women are making exercise and fitness a part of their lives. This is a very positive development. What is not such a positive step forward, however, is the sacrifice of menstrual health in order to pursue ever more exhausting and demanding training schedules.

Doctors are still not expressing enough concern about menstrual irregularity in female athletes. It is assumed that menstrual irregularity and being an athlete go together, but this is a dangerous assumption to make. Athletic amenorrhea is a potentially serious problem. It is associated with hormonal abnormalities that can lead to serious clinical consequences.

In the words of Dr. Carol Otis, chairperson of the American College of Sports Medicine Ad Hoc Task Force on Women's Issues in Sports Medicine, "Up until about the early 1980's, most of us regarded amenorrhea as a relatively benign condition and something that was a consequence of training. . . . Amenorrhea is a symptom of something going wrong. It is not a natural response of the female body to training. It is an indication of a potentially serious clinical problem" (quoted in Skolnick, "'Female Athlete Triad' Risk for Women").

Athletic menstrual dysfunction is not fully understood yet, but a number of theories are circulating at present about why female athletes are more prone to the condition than other women.

The first theory points to low body weight. During puberty, menses first occur when body-fat content rises above 17 percent, and menses cease when it falls below 12 percent. When body fat is too low to support a baby, the body is in a state of stress because it is malnourished, and so the hypothalamus does not send out signals to orchestrate the menstrual cycle. Many athletes, dancers, and gymnasts are below the 12 percent body-fat threshold and as a result are amenorrheaic.

Body fat and body weight do play a role in menstrual dysfunction, but perhaps not as significant a role as was once thought by experts. These factors do not explain, for example, why periods sometimes don't return when weight returns to normal. When this is the case, the absence of menstrual bleeding might be connected to the training schedule of the athlete and not to body fat.

Although increased training does often go hand-in-hand with a reduction in body fat, the indications are that an intense training schedule alters the menstrual cycle regardless of body fat. Experts such as Dr. P. T. Ellison, a Harvard anthropologist, have shown that energy expenditure is more likely to stop periods than to cause weight loss. The psychological and emotional stresses of strenuous exercise are associated with an increase in cortisol, which stimulates androgen production.

In the amenorrheaic athlete the adrenal gland may be secreting cortisol and androgen at near maximum levels even when the athlete is at rest. With high levels of stress hormones and androgens circulating, the ovaries will not be able to function properly.

POOR DIET

Disordered eating habits and poor nutrition place the body under stress, increasing the likelihood of androgen imbalance. If you have poor eating habits, sooner or later you will become deficient in certain vitamins and minerals essential to your body's mechanisms. The result is hormonal imbalance. Many women with poor eating habits also have menstrual irregularity. In order to cope with the distress caused by an inadequate intake of nutrients, the adrenal gland goes into overdrive and overproduces androgens. Sooner or later the ovaries will be affected and anovulation is likely. We will discuss diet further in chapter 5.

PROGESTERONE DEFICIENCY

If you are not ovulating you will also not be producing progesterone. While some of the effects of progesterone are uncomfortable—the bloating, cramping, nausea, and pain that accompany periods are caused by progesterone—its beneficial effects are many. In addition to preparing the body for pregnancy, progesterone contributes to bone density and thus helps to prevent later osteoporosis.

Progesterone also counteracts the effects of estrogen. If there is not enough progesterone, symptoms of estrogen dominance will occur. These include bloating, breast swelling, depression, weight gain, mood swings, irregular periods, diminished sex drive, tiredness, and water retention. Progesterone deficiency can also result in life-threatening conditions. The long-term medical risks of progesterone deficiency are heart disease and endometrial cancer caused by overstimulation of estrogen without progesterone.

A recent study at the Harvard School of Public Health and Center of Prevention of Cardiovascular Disease has come up with a possible connection between progesterone deficiency and heart disease. The area still needs greater study, but researchers working with heart cells found that the hormone inhibited the growth of smooth muscle cells on blood vessel walls, a condition which can contribute to clogged arteries, the precursors to heart attacks and strokes.

Progesterone prevents cancerous changes in the lining of the uterus that would otherwise result from estrogen. Without the continued stimulation of estrogen by progesterone, the endometrium can become abnormal and overgrown, resulting in a higher risk of cancer.

INFERTILITY

For five years now we have been trying to have a baby. I'm only twenty-nine, so I have got time, but I can't help worrying that there might be something wrong with me.

Linda, age twenty-nine

Last year was a depressing year. My husband and I were desperate to make a baby but nothing happened. I thought getting pregnant would be so easy. Well, it was for all my friends, but not for me. The thought that I might be infertile crosses my mind, but I keep pushing it away. It makes me feel so depressed.

Sarah, age thirty-six

Most women with PCOS or PCO experience temporary infertility. With treatment, fertility can return and conception is possible. In rare instances, when the ovaries become very diseased, the infertility is permanent.

There will come a time in every woman's life when she will have to decide if having a baby is an option or not. You may decide not to have children, but ideally you will have the opportunity to decide for yourself. If you have androgen disorder and anovulation, the decision is no longer yours; your hormones have decided for you. If no egg is released from the ovary, conception is impossible. You cannot get pregnant until the hormone problem is corrected and you start to ovulate again. Androgen disorder is robbing you not only of your ability to conceive but of your ability to chose to conceive when you want to.

You don't necessarily have to manifest other symptoms of androgen disorder to have PCOS or PCO and resulting infertility. So if you are having problems getting pregnant, androgen excess will be one of the first things your doctor checks you for.

According to Douglas, having an androgen problem does not usually result in irreversible fertility: "Women with PCO and PCOS are not irreversibly infertile, but the condition will make conception harder to achieve. In almost all cases, fertility will return with the correct hormonal treatment and conception is possible. However, if treatment is stopped, infertility usually returns."

In very rare cases of androgen disorder, infertility is indeed irreversible. Coming to terms with infertility is never easy. You will feel so many conflicting emotions all at once—anger, self-hatred, despair, confusion, dismay, disbelief—and above all an overwhelming sense of injustice, grief, and loss. Infertility is a crisis that affects all areas of your life. You need the love and support of family and friends, and in many cases therapy and counseling, to understand and accept the situation. In time you may come to realize that women can give birth in many ways apart from the biological. You are only infertile in the sense that childbirth is not an option, but in other areas of your life the opportunity for creativity and fulfillment still exists.

LIBIDO, SEXUAL ACTIVITY, AND MOOD

Some doctors vigorously assert that testosterone is crucially important for a normal sex drive in women, since it activates the brain's sexual circuits for both sexes. But this point is debatable, since many studies show little or no correlation between testosterone levels and a woman's sex drive.

Dr. Susan Rako (*The Hormone of Desire*) calls testosterone a female sex hormone. She argues that when women with low testosterone levels are given testosterone therapy, they often report feeling sexual again and more like their old selves. Rako believes that testosterone also enhances our psychological sense of well-being and that depression can actually be related to a deficiency in testosterone. It helps improve our sense of well-being and our energy level. Studies reveal that testosterone has a mood-lifting or antidepressant effect.

If this is the case, does it mean that the higher your androgen levels, the higher your sex drive and the better your mood?

No, says Rako. "It is interesting to note that women diagnosed with PCO syndrome who have blood levels of testosterone above the normal range have not been noted to experience increased libido" (p. 49).

Rako explains that if you are testosterone-deficient and are given testosterone therapy, your sex drive may improve, but raising the level of testosterone above normal levels does not increase sexual energy in women. High androgen levels in women do not automatically lead to an increased sexual desire and a sense of euphoria. Yes, testosterone will improve a woman's mood, but only when it is present in amounts that are normal. If testosterone levels rise above what is needed, women report not only hirsutism but insomnia, irritability, and nightmares. When the levels rise even higher, women can experience volatile mood shifts and aggression.

The crucial factor remains that of hormonal balance. You can feel your best only if your hormones are in balance.

SEXUAL ORIENTATION

When I began shaving my face three years ago and my periods stopped, I was apprehensive. Will men still find me attractive? Will I still be sexually aroused by them?

Sally, age thirty-seven

It is common these days, among both scientists and the general public, to believe that hormones explain sexual differences between men and women. Studies with rats have shown that the presence of an androgen such as testosterone in early life is critical for adult male sexual behavior, while its absence is essential for female behavior. Do our hormones then regulate our sexual behavior and choice of sexual partner?

Research into the hormonal regulation of sexual behavior in human beings is still in its infancy, and studies on humans are far less conclusive than those on rats. And the often-accepted notion that hormones dictate sexual behavior has been challenged by studies such as Anne Fausto-Sterling's *Myths of Gender*. Fausto-Sterling argues that studies of hormones and sex differences are often blinded by prejudice and bias. They encourage gender stereotyping. There is no conclusive proof that sexual orientation is hormonally based.

Yet the idea of male and female hormones is so deeply ingrained that many women with androgen disorder are concerned about the implications of high levels of male hormone on their sexual identity. Are they changing gender? Will their sexual preference change? Is the incidence of androgen disorder high among lesbians?

Dr. Geoffrey Redmond (*Women's Hormones*, p. 199) states that androgen excess may make a woman feel more inhibited because the symptoms can be embarrassing, but it will not affect her sex drive or change her sexual preference.

Androgen disorder can appear in any woman regardless of her age, background, race, or sexual orientation. Studies reveal that the number of lesbians with androgen disorder is not excessively high. But we really have no idea how many women with androgen disorder are lesbians, as many women who have the condition do not seek treatment. Women who do see a doctor often do so because of fertility problems, and at least in the past, these women have tended to be heterosexual.

Whatever her sexual orientation might be, the symptoms of androgen disorder can make any woman feel uncomfortable, embarrassed, and inhibited sexually. But an increase in androgen levels is unlikely to change sexual preference.

MOOD AND BEHAVIOR

Will high levels of androgen affect how a woman behaves, perhaps causing her to exhibit more so-called masculine traits of aggression and violence?

Studies on female athletes who use steroids and have very high testosterone levels seem to confirm that aggressive behavior increases significantly with increases in testosterone level. Excessive amounts of the hormone can even cause psychosis and violent behavior. One study conducted in 1985 by Strauss, Ligget, and Lanese revealed that eight out of ten women who increased their androgen levels felt more aggressive.

Dr. James M. Dabbs, Jr., a professor and researcher in the department of psychology at Georgia State University in Atlanta, came up with some important findings in the early 1990s. His studies showed not only that testosterone levels are highest in the morning for both men and women and that sexual experience stimulates testosterone production in women, but that sportsmen and high-profile lawyers have higher testosterone levels than those who are unemployed.

The conclusion Dabbs draws from all this, however, was not that high testosterone necessarily causes an aggressive personality but that to understand human nature you need to understand both biological and social forces. Behavioral or biological approaches to human behavior alone are incomplete. He states that testosterone may affect behavior but that the behavior itself also affects testosterone levels. How every woman responds to a rise in testosterone will be unique and according to her personality and social circumstances ("Salivary Testosterone Measurements," pp. 83–86).

In short, it is really impossible to draw any conclusions that apply to every woman. Rako makes a great point: "Popular belief about the relationship between testosterone and emotions and behavior has been limited to the correlation of higher testosterone levels with violence and aggression. This gross correlation in no way does justice to the complex of human issues involved in human emotions" (*Hormone of Desire*, p. 78).

All that can be said definitively at this moment is that when testosterone levels rise above normal in women they are still significantly lower than the levels in men. There are unlikely to be any behavioral changes. If anything at all, a woman with high testosterone levels might feel more assertive, but most women report feeling more irritable. The only case in which behavior might significantly be affected would be if androgen levels were dangerously high because of drug use or serious disease.

MENOPAUSE

In some women, the pituitary gland goes into overdrive at menopause and tries to get the ovaries to ovulate by producing more testosterone. For a short time androgen levels increase and the symptoms of androgen excess manifest themselves. For some the effects will be subtle, for others more dramatic. There may be changes in facial hair or changes in body fat, such as fat around the hips and buttocks suddenly moving upward to the waist, which is more typical of men. The cholesterol pattern may become similar to that of men.

Far more common than androgen excess at menopause is androgen deficiency. A declining testosterone level is an aspect of normal menopause and aging but, like estrogen deficiency at menopause, it can cause problems.

Androgen Deficiency

I feel terrible. I seem to have lost my sex drive altogether. I love my husband very much, but I just am not interested in sex anymore. My loss of libido makes me feel frustrated, and my husband thinks that I don't want him. I know that at menopause the libido can decline, but I did not think it would go altogether. What I wouldn't give to get some sexual spark back. In fact, come to think of it, what I wouldn't give to get some of my zest for life back. These days I feel despondent and lethargic.

Sometimes I wake up in the early hours of the morning and cry quietly to myself until the alarm goes off at seven.

Even then I lie in bed and think there is no point in getting up. I look back on my life and see only failure. There seems to be no light at the end of this tunnel of darkness.

Janet, age forty-nine

Typically it is during the three years prior to menopause and through the five years following that women notice symptoms of androgen deficiency, although androgen levels begin to decline gradually in women on average from the thirties onward.

As we approach menopause there is a natural decline in the production of the sex hormones estrogen and androgen. The term *androgen disorder* generally refers to an excessive androgen production and should not be applied to androgen deficiency at menopause. However, because the subject of androgen deficiency in women has been as neglected as the subject of androgen excess, I will discuss it briefly.

For most women, this gradual decline of androgen goes unnoticed. For others there will be a decrease in libido and sexual response. Women who are on androgen-lowering medications, such as the Pill, may also experience androgen deficiency symptoms. Recent research suggests that up to one-third of us could experience androgen deficiency during perimenopause.

We need our testosterone. It has many benefits. So when levels are low, how does that make us feel? What are the emotional and physical effects of the androgen deficiency that is most often experienced by women during perimenopause and menopause?

According to Rako (*Hormone of Desire*, p. 63), the most noticeable signs of androgen deficiency are a decrease in sexual desire and sense of well-being, lower energy levels, lessening of sexual responsiveness in the nipples, decreased ability to orgasm, and thinning of pubic hair. To this list could be added fatigue, loss of muscle tone, and lack of mental sharpness. Your skin and hair might become dry. You could lose muscle tone in the bladder and pelvis and experience urinary incontinence. There is an increased risk of developing osteoporosis. You will most likely feel a loss of interest in sex, perhaps feeling as if your sexual switches had been turned off.

If you experience any of these symptoms, you may feel sensitive and embarrassed about seeking medical advice. Why? Because of age-old assumptions about women's sexuality. A woman approaching menopause who complains of loss of libido, sparse pubic hair, and vaginal dryness is often not given the consideration she deserves. She will be told that this is just a part of getting old. The belief that when a woman's reproductive life is over she really has no need to feel sexual desire might underly the doctor's casual attitude and reluctance to offer treatment.

Loss of sexual desire is not automatic when you reach menopause. Many women enjoy satisfying sex lives at every stage of their lives. Many, however, will notice that they have a decline in libido at menopause, which may well be connected to low levels of androgen and other hormonal imbalances. When levels return to normal, many women report feeling renewed. They want and enjoy sex again.

A lower testosterone level is also one of the frequently neglected factors when it comes to the problem of fatigue at menopause. Depression that is hard to diagnose could also be caused by low levels of testosterone.

Although testosterone can be as beneficial as estrogen and progesterone to women at menopause, most doctors are still hesitant to prescribe androgen for loss of energy and libido. There is the fear of side effects, most notably the increased risk of heart disease. And there is the question of whether adding male hormone to estrogen replacement therapy diminishes estrogen's cardiac protection. It does seem that the addition of testosterone lowers the level of good cholesterol and increases the bad. There is also concern about a possible link between testosterone and liver damage.

Very little research has been done on the long-term effects of testosterone deficiency and how supplementary testosterone can improve a woman's quality of life at menopause. There is still no conclusive research to prove that androgens will increase a woman's libido, and many doctors believe that lack of interest in sex is never caused entirely by hormonal imbalance.

Without adequate information and advice from medical professionals, few women understand the role androgen plays in their lives at menopause, so most women are not in a position to make a decision about whether they should have this treatment. Many believe it will make them get acne or grow facial and body hair, or develop muscles and broad shoulders. The truth is that these symptoms occur only if testosterone is taken in excessive amounts. Women need to understand that a small but effective low dose of the hormone can be taken without the risk of side effects for a substantial period of time.

The final chapter in this section will explore the third group of clinically significant manifestations of androgen disorder: metabolic and systemic disturbances.

5

Metabolic and Systemic Disorders

he symptoms of androgen disorder primarily affect your appearance and your reproductive cycle. Unpleasant and uncomfortable as the symptoms are, they are not life-threatening. Left untreated for too long, however, androgen disorder is a severe health risk. In addition to causing infertility, it can cause metabolic changes that increase your risk of diabetes, hypertension, and heart disease. And it may also increase the risk of certain types of cancer. In this chapter we will take a look at these metabolic and systemic factors as they interact with androgen disorder.

HORMONES AND METABOLISM

I'm nearly fifty pounds overweight. I can't recall anything that triggered this weight gain. I have always eaten sensibly. The extra weight makes me feel tired and uncomfortable. I can't fit into any of the clothes I used to wear. I haven't had a period for nine months.

Linda, age thirty-nine

If only I could loose ten pounds. I'd feel so much better. I've tried dieting, exercise, but nothing seems to work.

Samantha, age thirty-one

I used to be so slim in my teens and twenties, and look at me now. I'm fifteen pounds too heavy. I really don't like the way I look.

Lauren, age thirty-four

Life is not fair. I eat the same as, perhaps even less than, my friends. I eat healthily and yet I just can't lose weight. What is wrong with me? I work out religiously and still the weight does not shift. Some days I just feel listless, unhappy, and hopeless about it all.

Mary, age thirty-six

Metabolism is the process of turning our food into energy for the body. *Enzymes* are biological catalysts that regulate all chemical reactions that make up the metabolic pathways. Life is therefore a process directed by enzymes. Many doctors believe that androgen imbalance interferes with the work of digestive enzymes and causes metabolic changes.

The rate of metabolism is the rate at which calories from food are burned up. Every woman's metabolic rate is unique to her. This explains why it is futile to compare your weight gain with that of other women. Your friend may be able to eat all she wants and never gain weight, while you put on weight when you are on a diet.

If your metabolism is efficient, food will be burned up quickly. If your metabolism is slow, you will tend to put on weight more easily. Most of us have some idea of what our metabolic rate is:

- If you are highly active and losing weight is easy for you, you have a fast metabolic rate.

- If you enjoy moderate exercise and lose weight slowly, you have a moderate metabolic rate.

- If you don't enjoy exercise and find weight loss difficult, your metabolic rate is slow.

Your metabolic rate can be affected by a number of factors. Stress is one of them. The adrenal cortex produces hormones to reduce stress. It also controls carbohydrate, protein, mineral, salt, and waste metabolism. If your adrenal gland is working overtime to counteract stress, it will become exhausted and overproduce androgen, which slows down your metabolic rate. Underactive thyroid glands, high insulin, and high blood sugar levels will also make your food burn slowly.

When your metabolism is slow, you feel lethargic and tired. You gain weight quickly. You may also crave sweet foods, processed carbohydrates, and starchy foods. You are likely to have poor circulation and dry skin.

Is slow metabolism and hormonal imbalance then to blame for weight gain that can't be explained? Many doctors believe that these two factors can sufficiently explain why some people have such difficulty loosing weight. However, before you stoically accept that you have not only a slow metabolism but also a hormonal imbalance that makes weight loss impossible without the help of drugs, remember that there is still no real proof that these factors determine weight gain. There are doctors who firmly believe that metabolic rate and hormones are not the causes of weight gain but that it is almost always caused by eating more food than the body needs for its daily activity and maintenance.

As is so often the case with two extreme points of view, the truth probably lies somewhere in between. If you are having trouble loosing weight and you don't really understand why, consider all the alternatives. Think about hormonal treatment, think about increasing your metabolic rate with exercise, and think about your diet.

DIABETES

If you have androgen disorder and anovulation, it is highly likely that you are insulin-resistant and at high risk of suffering from non-insulin-dependent diabetes (NIDDM), sometimes called adult-onset diabetes.

In America it is estimated that millions of people are diabetic but don't know it, because symptoms will appear only once the disease is fully established. Symptoms, when they occur, include tiredness and the need to pass urine frequently, especially during the night, blurred vision, and a craving for large amounts of liquid.

The underlying cause of adult-onset diabetes is the body's inability to effectively use the vital hormone insulin. Insulin is essential for processing sugar into the energy needed by the body's vital organs and tissues. A diet consisting of too many simple sugars and processed carbohydrates is thought to cause insulin resistance after a while. The body just becomes less sensitive to insulin, and increasingly large amounts of the hormone is needed to process sugar.

Insulin resistance is believed to be one of the reasons overweight people have problems losing weight. In many overweight women, the insulin that is produced never reaches the correct receptors in the cells. Sometimes there may also be too few insulin receptors to allow the glucose to enter and be used for fuel. The result is high blood sugar levels, hormonal confusion, and a very slow metabolic rate.

The connection between insulin regulation and androgen problems is a new area of research in which much is still to be learned. A 1998 study at the Medical College of Virginia Hospitals in Richmond found that women with polycystic ovary syndrome ovulate more frequently when their insulin levels are lowered with medication (*American Health for Women*, p. 20).

Diabetes and androgen disorder do appear to be related. This may be due to the interconnection between blood sugar hormones, stress hormones, and sex hormones that Ann Louise Gittleman stresses in *Before the Change*. When the body can't utilize insulin effectively, the ovary reacts unusually by making too much testosterone. So women with diabetes are likely to have androgen imbalance, and vice versa.

According to Tori Hudson, N.D. (*Women's Health Update*), "It is estimated that women with PCOS account for at least 10% of all cases of glucose intolerance in premenopausal women. Diabetes develops earlier in women with PCOS, in the 20s and 30s, than in the general population (50s and 60s)."

An androgen disorder could be an early warning sign of the possibility of diabetes developing. So do make sure you take steps to prevent this. You should find out if you are insulin-resistant, or if you have impaired glucose tolerance, which means higher than normal blood sugar levels.

WEIGHT GAIN

Women with androgen disorder often tend to be overweight. Is obesity then a cause of androgen disorder? Or does androgen disorder cause obesity?

According to Dr. James Douglas, "The answer to this is rather like the chicken and the egg. Which came first: the excess androgen that caused the weight gain, or does the weight gain make an androgen problem more likely?"

There are both thin and overweight women with androgen disorder, but it is believed that obesity is a contributory factor. Some doctors think that weight gain causes androgen disorder. The higher the weight, the harder it is for a woman to ovulate. Obesity causes an increase in insulin, which stimulates the ovaries to make more androgen. Some studies show that overweight women are more likely to have androgen disorder than women within the normal weight range. Other doctors believe that excess androgens cause metabolic changes that make weight gain very likely.

A patient with androgen disorder will find it hard to lose weight. When testosterone levels are high, the body tends to retain fluid and hold body fat. Many women with PCOS have tried a dozen or so crash diets. There will be an initial weight loss, and then the body will resist any further weight loss and hit a plateau. These women will feel discouraged and gain back the pounds lost. In addition to this, testosterone also has an anabolic effect on the metabolism: it will increase the appetite.

This is not to say that every woman with an androgen disorder is overweight. Studies of women with hirsutism show that sufferers do have a higher than average body weight and problems with cholesterol, but they also show that many women with androgen disorder are slender. We still don't really understand why one woman gains weight while another does not. Research just indicates that excess androgens could be a contributory factor. Douglas believes that circumstances vary from person to person. Each case will be different, but there is no doubt that more often than not weight gain and androgen disorder go hand-in-hand.

If you are overweight there may be no simple solution. Sometimes dieting and exercising just don't work, however hard you try. In addition to diet and exercise, hormonal causes, the way you metabolize food, your environment, and genetics may all play a part. The best way to treat weight gain is to acknowledge that it is a complex condition that rarely has an easy solution.

FLUID RETENTION

If your androgen levels are high, you are likely to retain fluid. Testosterone is anabolic. It will make the body form new tissue, and to do this the body must retain water and sodium. If fluid retention is extreme, the hands, wrists, feet, and ankles will swell and the face and hands may become puffy.

Feeling swollen and bloated is distressing and uncomfortable. It can make you feel anxious, heavy, and even mildly depressed.

HYPERTENSION

Doctors are recognizing that there is a tendency to high blood pressure in women who have androgen disorder, particularly those who are overweight. Women with high blood pressure also often have insulin resistance and diabetes. According to Dr. Geoffrey Redmond, "High blood pressure is not a female problem in itself. However, hypertension is as common in some women as in men and can be associated with androgen disorders" (*Women's Hormones*, p. 381).

High blood pressure is a frightening problem because it can creep up on you like a thief in the night. You may not know that you have it, because there are often no symptoms. So if you have androgen disorder, it is important that you find out not only if you have diabetes but also if you have high blood pressure.

Why is high blood pressure so dangerous? Because over the years it can cause the heart to enlarge and wear itself out, eventually causing heart failure when the heart can no longer pump blood throughout the body. The arteries have to bear too much pressure over the years and gradually get damaged. One day they might burst and cause a stroke in the brain. Coronary heart disease may also result. Excessive pressure on the arteries can also cause the arteries to narrow and cut off the blood supply to the heart. In short, hypertension can slowly destroy your circulatory system.

HEART DISEASE

I know I have a problem and I should loose weight. Last year my doctor told me that my cholesterol profile indicated that

I could be at risk of heart disease. I worry about it a lot but just can't seem to stick to a diet.

Monica, age forty-one

Some doctors believe that hormonal factors are very important in the development of heart disease in women. Excess testosterone causes metabolic changes in your body. It is thought that it increases the amount of bad cholesterol in your body and decreases the amount of good cholesterol.

A poor cholesterol profile is a high risk factor for heart disease. A high percentage of women with this risk factor will get heart disease.

Heart disease is the most common cause of death in women. It kills many more women than breast cancer and far more women than men. If you have androgen disorder, it is of vital importance that you become aware that the condition may eventually affect your cardiovascular health.

ENDOMETRIAL CANCER

Women with PCO are not producing enough progesterone hormone. Without progesterone, the lining of the womb, or endometrium, can become abnormal and, if left untreated, cancerous. This condition takes many years to develop, but eventually it can prove fatal. It can be prevented, however, by seeking treatment early enough. That is why irregular periods, whether absent or heavy and prolonged, should never be ignored.

BREAST CANCER

Obese women with high androgen levels are at increased risk of breast cancer. Two out of three breast tumors seem to be stimulated by estrogen, progesterone, or prolactin. Excess androgens convert to estrogen in fat tissue.

OVARIAN CANCER

Women who suffer from PCO and PCOS are at higher risk of abnormal cell development in the ovaries, which can lead to ovarian cancer.

LIVER DAMAGE

Nothing has as yet been proved for women, but studies in men indicate that testosterone is linked to liver disease.

Androgen disorder is a serious medical condition that needs to be treated. The signs and symptoms are unpleasant and disturbing both physically and emotionally. Androgen disorder gradually injures the body, and can lead eventually to severe health complications. The good news is that the condition can be easily treated. In fact, according to Redmond (*Women's Hormones*), androgen disorders are the easiest of hormonal disorders to treat.

If you think you have some of the signs and symptoms of androgen disorder, you could well be suffering from a medical condition that needs treatment. Don't just put up with a state of poor health. Go to see your doctor. Find out if you have some kind of hormonal imbalance. Think about the long-term health risks of neglecting these symptoms.

Should you be diagnosed with some form of androgen imbalance, you will need to make decisions about the kind of treatment you want. The next section of this book will focus on prevention, self-help, and the ways doctors of both conventional and alternative medicine treat the disorder.

Part 3

Prevention, Self-Help, and Treatment

6

How to Help Yourself

Since the 1950s, millions of women have been treated with hormones by their doctors. These hormones alter and modify our biological functions or attempt to correct hormonal deficiency or excess. Many of us, despite the proven success record of hormonal therapy, are still reluctant to undergo hormonal therapy. We would like to explore other alternatives. Our doctors, however, often don't consider what our preferences are. Hormonal therapy works, so hormonal therapy is prescribed, even for those who are reticent about taking it.

Fear of side effects is the usual complaint when hormonal therapy is advised. We are right to be concerned here. Each form of hormonal therapy carries with it certain risks. The Pill is the most frequently prescribed form. Not only can it cause nausea, possible weight gain, and mood swings, but it totally abolishes the normal menstrual cycle, distorts metabolism, and may cause blood clots, infertility, and birth defects. Another drawback of hormonal replacement therapy is that it is not short term: you take it for life.

When we take artificial hormones, we are walking about in an altered biochemical state. Sir Charles Dodds, the British scientist who synthesized orally effective estrogen in 1938, lived to deplore the application of his discovery. "When a clock is working," he said glumly, "you don't tinker with it" (quoted in Seaman, *Women and the Crisis in Sex Hormones*, xii).

The casual prescription of hormones for women is certainly to be deplored. It is all too often used by doctors as a quick-fix remedy when other less harsh measures might be equally effective.

The term *hormonal therapy* carries with it the implication of a disease that needs to be treated. But menopause and infertility, the most common conditions for which hormones are prescribed, are not diseases. If your doctor is advising hormonal therapy for these conditions, you should certainly have your reservations and consider all options, including safe alternatives, before you make your decision.

An androgen disorder, however, is not like menopause. It is not a natural state for the female body to be in. There is a strong case for arguing that it does merit hormonal therapy. Sure, there are risks attached, but often the benefits will outweigh the risks.

There are ways you can help yourself if you have been diagnosed with androgen disorder. But you will have to make the decision that you really want to make changes to improve your lifestyle and health. Although in most cases hormonal therapy from your doctor is still the only proven therapy, there are several natural methods that have been shown to have the potential to change the course of androgen imbalance. These changes come under the headings of diet, exercise, and stress management.

Changing the way you live is one of the hardest things to do. We all get stuck in routines and habits, but if you really want to feel better, this is the challenge you have to face. You will need a lot of patience: sometimes feeling better may take months or even years. You will also need a lot of motivation and willpower. Taking drugs given by your doctor provides a quicker, easier alternative, but bear in mind that even if you are prescribed hormonal therapy by your doctor, he or she will still strongly recommend that you try to cultivate a healthy lifestyle to complement your treatment.

After discussing diet, exercise, and stress management, we will turn to suggestions for managing the specific symptoms of androgen imbalance.

DIET: UNDERSTANDING THE BASICS OF GOOD NUTRITION

In the words of Ann Louise Gittleman, "Diet, hormones and the presence or absence of many female symptoms are all interconnected. It may be many years before researchers have worked out all the intricate and marvelous interactions of blood sugar, stress and ovarian hormone and how these interactions differ from woman to woman" (*Before the Change*, p. 40).

Many doctors and nutritionists like Gittleman believe that what we eat will affect the hormonal balance in our bodies. If we don't eat a balanced diet, we miss out on nutrients. Without proper nutrients, the body can't manufacture the hormones it needs to function normally.

Women with androgen disorder need to eat a diet that focuses on keeping their hormones in balance. The best way to do this is to make sure your diet has the correct amount of nutrients. Nutrients are substances in food that help the body grow, repair, and sustain itself.

There are six classes of nutrients: carbohydrates, proteins, fats, vitamins, minerals, and water. Carbohydrates, proteins, and fats are used by your body as a source for energy. Your body does not get energy from vitamins and minerals, but they are essential because they help various bodily processes and chemical reactions to take place. For instance, magnesium is an important player in the process of releasing energy from the food you eat. Finally, water is the medium in which all your bodily reactions take place. Water makes up 60 percent of our body, and without water we could not live.

Knowing what foods contain which nutrients and what is important for a hormonally regulated diet will help you plan a balanced diet. Your diet needs to be composed of a balance of carbohydrates, proteins, and fats with the correct intake of vitamins, minerals, and water. A stable blood sugar level is one of the benefits of a balanced diet. When your blood sugar levels are normal you will have more energy, concentrate better, feel more relaxed and happy, and generally feel healthier. In addition, you will be less likely to have hormonal problems.

Proteins

Proteins are the substances that build tissues for growth and repair. They also help to reduce menstrual problems. If you don't get enough protein in your diet, your body will break down its own muscle tissue. The result is loss of muscle tone, thinning hair, food cravings, and fatigue. Proteins also stabilize blood sugar levels by stimulating glucagon, which restores blood sugar levels and releases fat. Increased amounts of protein will increase metabolic rate significantly, help burn fat, and give you more energy. Proteins are found in foods like lean meat, poultry, foul, fish, eggs, milk and milk products, beans, nuts, yeast, grains, soy, and wheat germ. Protein should account for about 20 to 30 percent of a healthy diet.

Carbohydrates and Fiber

Carbohydrates, our main source of energy, are found in starch, sugar, and fiber. Far too many women with hormonal problems eat too much carbohydrate. In recent years the emphasis has for too long been on diets high in carbohydrates and low in fat. The standard recommendation has been for 70 percent of your diet to be from carbohydrates. The trouble with this is that carbohydrates not converted immediately by the body into sugar and used are stored as fat. A high-carbohydrate diet should be avoided if you suffer from hormone imbalance.

It is very important to eat the right kinds and amounts of carbohydrates in a hormonally regulated diet. Starch is a good source of carbohydrates, and it is found in bread, potatoes, rice, pasta, fruit, vegetables, and cereal. Sugars are not a good source of carbohydrates if they are found in sucrose (table sugar), but natural sugars, found in fruits and vegetables, are fine. Fiber provides little energy, but is very important because it plays an important part in regular bowel movements. Good sources are whole-meal bread and pasta, vegetables, and fruit. Opinions differ, but many nutritionists now think that foods containing starch and fiber should make up about 40 to 50 percent of your diet.

Fats

Fats keep the body functions working, and it is thought that they should account for about 30 percent of our diet. As we need fat to produce hormones, it is obvious what the dangers of a very low fat diet are for women with androgen problems. Fat is essential for women with hormonal imbalance, but far too many of us eat a low-fat diet in the misguided belief that it will help us lose weight. The truth is that we need a certain amount of fat in our bodies to burn and metabolize fat. Saturated fats are mainly of animal origin and are found in meat, milk, butter, cheese, soy oil, olive oil, and nuts. They should be taken in moderation as they can raise blood cholesterol to dangerous levels. Polyunsaturated and monounsaturated fats have greater health benefits. They tend to occur in plants, and they lower blood cholesterol. Other good sources are fish and seaweed, flaxseed oil, green leafy vegetables, liver, olive oil, and soy oil.

Vitamins

- Vitamin A fights infection and prevents dry skin and poor bone growth. It is found in vegetables, milk, butter, margarine, and egg yolks.

- Thiamin is important for carbon dioxide removal during respiration. It is found in whole-grain nuts and seeds.

- Riboflavin is needed for growth and is found in milk, meat, eggs, and leafy vegetables.

- Niacin helps to prevent disease, improve the mood, and promote a glowing complexion. You can find it in milk, eggs, cheeses, and fish.

- Pantothenic acid is essential for energy metabolism and is found in many foods such as meat, fish, poultry, whole grain cereals, and dried beans.

- Vitamin B6 is important for the metabolism of proteins. It is found in spinach, broccoli, and bananas.

- Vitamin B12 promotes healthy skin and helps maintain a healthy nervous system. It is found in meat, milk, eggs, cheese, and fish.

- Biotin is important for carbohydrate and fat metabolism. It is found in liver, peanuts, and cheese.

- Folate promotes cell production and healthy skin and is found in leafy green vegetables, chicken, liver, and kidneys.

- Vitamin C, found in green vegetables and citrus fruits, prevents colds, heals wounds, and is essential for normal metabolism and the reduction of menstrual problems. The adrenal glands absorb more vitamin C than any other part of the body. This vitamin boosts the immune system and protects us from toxins.

- Vitamin D, good for bone growth and calcium absorption, is also an aid in alleviating menstrual difficulties and is found in tuna fish, eggs, butter, and cheese.

- Vitamin E promotes blood clotting and is found in milk, vegetables, liver, rice, and bran.

- Vitamin K is active in maintaining the involuntary nervous system, vascular system, and involuntary muscles. It is found in wheat germ, vegetable oil, and whole-grain breads and cereals.

Minerals

- Calcium prevents blood clotting and is necessary for bone growth, healthy teeth, and iron absorption, as well as being an aid in relieving menstrual problems. It is found in milk, milk products, egg yolks, green vegetables, and shellfish.

- Copper is an aid in the metabolism of iron and is found in liver and whole grains.

- Florin strengthens teeth and is found in fluorinated water and tea.

- Iron is the basic component of blood hemoglobin and prevents anemia. It is found in meat, green vegetables, yeast, and wheat germ.

- Iodine is found in seafood and seaweed and is an aid in regulating energy use in the body. It is found in seaweed and seafood.

- Magnesium, found in milk, grains, vegetables, fruits, and cereals, is involved in the normal functioning of the brain, spinal cord, and nerves and is an aid in forming bones and alleviating menstrual problems.

- Potassium is needed for healthy nerves and muscles and is found in milk, fruit, and vegetables.

- Sodium helps maintain adequate water in cells in the body and is found in table salt, milk, and meat.

- Phosphorus found in milk, yogurt, yeast, and wheat germ is required for bone growth, strong teeth, and energy transformation.

- Zinc plays an essential role in the development of reproductive organs and in the body's enzyme systems. It is found in egg yolks, milk, nuts, peas, and beans.

Water

Our bodies are made up of about two-thirds water, so the intake and distribution of fluid is important for all hormonal systems. If the body is deprived of water, blood volume is reduced and the blood does not circulate to the tissues as effectively. The brain is most affected; you might even feel dizzy if you are dehydrated, and you will almost certainly feel fatigued. The solution is to drink enough water—six to eight glasses a day is the recommended amount.

Further Recommendations

Reducing or eliminating the amount of caffeine and alcohol is important not only for a balanced, healthy diet but for women who suffer from hormonal problems. Alcohol can cause high blood pressure and caffeine can cause stress, fatigue, headaches, and lack of energy. Caffeine and alcohol also deplete the body of water and minerals because they have a diuretic effect. Cigarettes and drugs are also damaging, and they can become addictive.

The timing of meals is significant. Sometimes eating three meals a day will not suit you, and you will feel better having frequent light snacks to avoid hypoglycemia, which occurs when the body goes from the fed to the fasting state. When food is spread out over the day with light, regular snacking, your body can make better use of calories, and you will feel energized because you have a constant supply of energy.

How Much Should I Eat Each Day?

Food guides can not only help you assess the nutritional quality of your diet but also help you determine if you are eating too much or too little. Remember, though, that they are not perfect, and as scientists discover new information, food guides change and nutritionists revise their opinions. The following are the current recommendations:

- Bread, rice, cereal, and pasta: six to eleven servings a day

- Fruit: two to four servings a day

- Vegetables: three to five servings a day

- Milk, yogurt, and cheese: two to three servings a day

- Meat, poultry, fish, eggs, and nuts: two to three servings a day

- Fats, oils, and sweets: to be eaten sparingly

A balanced diet should contain the right quality and quantity of food for you. How much you need will depend on your build and how active you are. Height and weight charts (see figure 6) can give you only a vague idea of your ideal weight for your height. They are typically based on data from people who buy life insurance, not on statistics from the general population. Don't get too anxious if your natural weight does not match the weight charts that your doctor or insurance company gives you. These charts do not address the biological variability among women and the fact that sometimes your body knows what its natural weight should be.

The weight that is right for you may also fluctuate on a daily basis and with the seasons. One of the best things you can do when trying to lose weight for health reasons is to throw away the

Height (in.)	Weight (lbs.)			
	Underweight	Normal	Overweight	Obese
57	101	102–133	134–150	151
58	103	104–136	137–153	154
59	106	107–140	141–157	158
60	107	108–142	143–159	160
61	110	111–145	146–164	165
62	113	114–149	150–168	169
63	115	116–152	153–172	173
64	118	119–156	157–176	177
65	121	122–160	161–180	181
66	123	124–163	164–184	185
67	126	127–167	168–188	189
68	129	130–170	171–192	193
69	132	133–174	175–196	197
70	134	135–178	179–200	201

Fig. 6. Weight for Height Values (Medium Build)

scale. Try to trust your instincts more. Eat a nutritious diet and exercise more. Let how you feel be the guide. Focus on your health, exercise levels, and diet rather than your body weight.

Some of us gain weight for emotional reasons, but many of us just have bigger bodies than the abnormally thin models we see in magazines. Our natural weight may just not correspond to the unhealthy cultural ideal of thinness that we see every day. We all have to make peace with our weight at some time in our lives, and this involves accepting our natural body size. You will know what your natural weight is, because it is the weight at which you feel most comfortable, healthy, and energetic.

Should I Take a Vitamin and Mineral Supplement?

In an ideal world you would get all the nutrients you need from the food you eat, have good digestion, never get stressed out, and never lose a night's sleep. Unfortunately, nobody lives in this ideal world. Therefore, taking a vitamin and mineral supplement that reflects the recommended dietary allowances (RDAs) guidelines should be a part of your daily nutrient routine. A combination vitamin and mineral supplement is advisable for women with androgen disorder. Separate vitamin and mineral supplements can also be taken when necessary.

As always, when taking any form of supplement, make sure you check that what you are taking is safe. You might consider getting advice from a doctor, dietitian, or nutritionist.

Nutrients and the Adrenal Glands

An exhausted adrenal gland is associated with androgen disorder and high levels of stress. Optimal stress management is dependent on optimal adrenal function. Some diet recommendations can help the adrenal gland and supply it with what it needs to function optimally.

Vitamin B5 (pantothenic acid) serves as a major energy source for the adrenal glands; therefore, deficiency of B5 can lead to adrenal exhaustion. B5 is important because it helps in the production and release of adrenal hormones from the adrenal gland, which help counteract stress and which control carbohydrate, protein, mineral, salt, and water metabolism. B5 is found in eggs, fish, meat, poultry, blue cheese, whole grains, lentils, corn, peas, sweet potatoes, green beans, and sunflower seeds.

Other B vitamins are also important for healthy adrenal glands, especially B2 and B5. The best way to get the benefits of vitamin B is by eating whole grains and legumes. B6 will also relieve some of the symptoms of water retention and bloating, skin eruptions, and mood swings. Foods that contain B6 include soybeans, spinach, and bananas. Most nutritionists agrees that the best way to take B vitamins is in B-complex form rather than separately, because the B vitamins affect one another's metabolism.

Vitamin C is especially valuable to women suffering from hormonal imbalance and adrenal gland exhaustion. Fruits and vegetables are the main source. Vitamin E is also important, as it is an essential nutrient for the production of hormones. Foods high in vitamin E include green leafy vegetables, sunflower oil, and whole-wheat flour.

Green vegetables, such as broccoli, and yellow and orange vegetables, such as sweet potatoes and fruit, are rich in many minerals consumed by a stressed adrenal gland. Brewer's yeast, brown rice, legumes, nuts, olive oil, seeds, wheat germ, and whole grains are healthy additions to the diet as well.

Include in your diet deep-water ocean fish, salmon or tuna, garlic, and onions to boost the immune system. Avoid alcohol, caffeine, and tobacco, as these substances are toxic to the adrenal glands. Stay away from excess fats, fried foods, ham, pork, highly processed foods, red meats, sodas, sugars, and white flour. These put unnecessary stress on the adrenal glands.

Sea vegetables contain zinc, manganese, chromium, magnesium, potassium, phosphorus, and iodine. Zinc and manganese are especially important for the adrenal glands. Zinc is needed in all metabolic functions. You can find zinc and manganese in sea vegetables, nuts, seeds, and lean beef.

Best Diet Choice for Androgen Disorder

Nutritional improvement and regular exercise are very powerful ways to improve your health. You may be amazed at how much better you feel when you start eating a balanced diet and stop making unhealthy food choices. Studies have shown that a diet high in fat is linked to disease in the female organs—so watch your fat intake and increase the amount of fiber you eat. It is believed that 60 percent of all cancers in women are related to dietary fat and high estrogen levels. Many women with androgen disorder have elevated estrogen levels, so a diet that is high in fiber and sensible in its fat intake would be beneficial. Don't eliminate fat from your diet altogether, though; just avoid too much saturated fat. Vegetable fiber has the ability to improve the metabolism of estrogen in the intestine so that less estrogen can circulate in the bloodstream. According to Dr. Christiane Northrup, a "low fat, mostly vegetarian, low or no dairy, high fiber diet can significantly relieve polycystic ovary syndrome, promote your natural body weight, improve emotional well-being and reduce the risk of breast, ovarian, and uterine cancer and heart disease" (*Women's Bodies*, p. 592).

Dietary recommendations to prevent acne include eating a low-fat, low-sugar diet and avoiding milk. The hormones that are found it milk are thought to irritate acne.

Should I Try to Lose Weight?

If you have an androgen disorder and are overweight, weight loss will almost certainly be a part of the treatment program recommended by your doctor. Weight loss won't be easy if your weight gain is caused by a hormonal imbalance. However, androgen disorder shouldn't be used as an excuse not to start a healthy diet and exercise program.

As long as it is not taken to extremes, most women feel less stressed when their weight is manageable. Being seriously over- or underweight is one of the major causes of stress and low self-esteem among women. If you want to get some idea of how healthy your weight is for your height, the Body Mass Index (BMI) gives a more sophisticated height-weight correlation than the weight charts. To figure out your BMI, multiply your weight in pounds by seven hundred. Then divide this number by the square of your height in inches.

If this all sounds a bit too complicated, have a look at the BMI chart in figure 7. If your BMI is below 19, you are too thin. Between 19 and 25 is perfect, and you should maintain your body weight through healthy diet and exercise. If your BMI is between

Height

Body Weight

Height	19	20	21	22	23	24	25	26	27	28	29	30	31
4'10"	91	96	100	105	110	115	119	124	129	134	138	143	148
4'11"	94	99	104	109	114	119	124	128	133	138	143	148	153
5'	97	102	107	112	118	123	128	133	138	143	148	153	158
5'1"	100	106	111	116	122	127	132	137	143	148	153	158	164
5'2"	104	109	115	120	126	131	136	142	147	153	158	164	169
5'3"	107	113	118	124	130	135	141	146	152	158	163	169	175
5'4"	110	116	122	128	134	140	145	151	157	163	169	174	180
5'5"	114	120	126	132	138	144	150	156	162	168	174	180	186
5'6"	118	124	130	136	142	148	155	161	167	173	179	186	192
5'7"	121	127	134	140	146	153	159	166	172	178	185	191	198
5'8"	125	131	138	144	151	158	164	171	177	184	190	197	203
5'9"	128	135	142	149	155	162	169	176	182	189	196	203	209
5'10"	132	139	146	153	160	167	174	181	188	195	202	209	216
5'11"	136	143	150	157	165	172	179	186	193	200	208	215	222
6'	140	147	154	162	169	177	184	191	199	206	213	221	228
Your BMI	19	20	21	22	23	24	25	26	27	28	29	30	31
	Optimal Weight							Overweight					

Fig. 7. **BMI Rating**

26 to 29, your weight is too high. It might be a good idea to start exercising regularly and cutting back on fat and total calories, especially if your BMI is over 35. If your BMI is over 30, you are considered clinically obese. There are serious health risks associated with obesity, such as high blood pressure, heart disease, and diabetes. It is recommended that you slowly lose at least 10 percent of your body weight.

Being around your ideal weight for your height, age, and build is an essential part of a balanced, healthy lifestyle. If you are overweight, your risk of androgen disorder is significantly higher than that of a woman with a similar build. If you have an androgen disorder and are overweight, weight loss should be part of your recovery program.

There are hundreds of programs designed to help you lose weight. Some promise miracle results in short periods of time. Each of them has a different approach to the problem. The truth, though, is that there is no one solution that will work for everyone. A method of weight loss that works for one person may not work for you. You have to find what suits you, but in the end, if you want to lose weight in a safe, effective manner, the following diet rules always apply:

1. Lose weight slowly. Statistics prove that drastic weight loss is seldom effective and usually dangerous. Aim for a loss of a pound or so a week. A good weight-loss program makes sure you lose weight gradually and do not see it go on again when you stop.
2. Increase your activity levels. Basically, move about more. A regular program of exercise is best, if you can manage it.
3. Reduce the number of calories that you eat, and eat healthily. Losing weight safely and effectively is a matter of burning up more energy (calories) than we use. Energy comes from what we eat or drink. So the only really effective way to lose weight is to eat less.

4. Avoid foods full of saturated fat and sugar. Saturated fat is found in meat and dairy products. To cut down on saturated fat:

    • Drink skimmed milk.

    • Eat lean meat or remove all extra fat.

    • Eat more fish and poultry.

    • Limit the number of eggs you eat to three or four a week.

    • Eat butter in moderation.

    • Avoid cheese, cream cakes, chips, and pastries.

    • Use olive oil, vegetable oil, and sunflower oil.

    • Avoid sugar, cookies, and chocolate. Sugar turns to fat if it is not burned for energy.

    • Increase the amount of fiber in your diet.

    • Avoid too much salt, since it can lead to high blood pressure.

Should I Count Calories?

For many years now, women have been slaves to calorie counting. You go on a diet and restrict yourself to a certain number of calories a day. Statistics show that women of moderate activity levels need around two thousand calories a day and that this number decreases with age You do your best to try and keep within the range. The problem with dieting in this way is that it just does not work. It is restrictive and it takes the enjoyment out of eating.

All calories are not created equal. Knowing how many calories a certain food has tells you nothing about its nutritional value. For example, a chocolate bar may have three hundred calories. So you could eat five chocolate bars in one day and nothing else, making a total of fifteen hundred calories. This is a low-calorie diet, but nutritionally this food choice is a disaster, and long-term weight loss will not occur. Why? Because a chocolate bar cannot give your body the nutrients that it needs to metabolize fat and give you energy, health, and vitality.

The advice is to stop calorie counting and eat more nutritious foods. You should try to avoid foods that you know have little nutritional value. Eating one thousand calories of cake, popcorn, ice cream, and chips is vastly different from eating one thousand calories of whole grains, fish, fruits, and vegetables.

If you are determined to count calories and want to know how much you should be eating, you need to determine your metabolic rate. Determining the rate at which you burn up food can be done accurately only in a hospital, but the following is a simple, although rough, guide:

Add a zero to your weight in pounds.

Add your body weight to this value.

Example: 130-pound woman:

1,300 + 130 = 1,630 calories a day.

To loose weight you, would need to eat less than the amount arrived at using this formula. To do so, you would have to reduce your food intake and increase your activity levels.

Many dieters make the mistake of skipping meals. If you want to loose weight, you need to keep your metabolic rate high. Breaking down food requires energy and increases your metabolic rate. When you skip meals or restrict your diet too much, you burn fewer calories and your body adjusts its metabolic rate so that you burn the food you do eat at an even slower rate.

What if I Have Diabetes?

If you are diabetic, being overweight can prevent insulin from actively working in your body. The usual advice for diabetics is to stick to a healthy natural diet with plenty of fresh fruit and vegetables, lean meats, and saturated fats. A high-carbohydrate diet used to be recommended for diabetics, but now researchers are coming to the view that a diet rich in monounsaturated fat may be better than a high-carbohydrate diet because it can lower blood sugar and maintain healthy levels of "good" fats in the bloodstream. Diabetics should avoid very low calorie diets, such as those that recommend milkshakes or powders to replace meals. Despite the claims of advertisers, such diets can lead to a loss of valuable nutrients.

Losing weight is recommended by all doctors if you are overweight and diabetic. In the early part of the nineteenth century, diabetics were put on starvation rations. Today the approach is a little more moderate. Diabetics should eat at least three meals a day, including breakfast, and eat a wide variety of nutritious foods.

Diabetics need to be especially careful to watch their saturated fat, sugar, and salt intake. They should also be careful of vitamin and mineral supplements, as there is evidence that high levels of some vitamins, such as vitamin C, can be harmful to diabetics. Sugar need not be avoided altogether, but it must be carefully controlled. The glycemic response is the way blood sugar levels rise in response to different foods. Diabetics must control their diet using the glycemic index, which gives a figure for each type of food, so that they can monitor closely their blood sugar levels in response to the food they eat. Diabetics need not give up alcohol altogether, but too much alcohol can be dangerous.

Diabetic foods should be avoided at all costs. In 1992 the British Diabetic Association issued a report condemning diabetic foods such as jam, chocolate, and biscuits. They are expensive, and in the words of the diabetic association, "in terms of composition, diabetic foods remain an outmoded relic from an era of carbohydrate avoidance."

EXERCISE

Diet is not the only factor that can affect the state of hormonal balance in your body: exercise can, too. One of the most effective ways to improve your health is by exercising, as long as you do not take it to the extreme. Too much exercise can have a disastrous effect on menstrual function, as we saw in chapter 4. A moderate amount of exercise, however, is beneficial. It should be a top priority at any age. Exercise improves circulation, helps maintain heart health, and lowers blood glucose. Aerobic activity reduces insulin and elevates glycagon. Exercise can trigger a release in the number of insulin receptors, mainly in muscle cells. Anaerobic exercise causes the body to secrete human growth hormone. Exercise can help us keep our heart and lungs in good condition, improve circulation, promote energy and health, remove toxic substances from the body, improve posture, and improve self-image. It can also delay the effects of aging and give you more energy.

Exercise is also helpful in reducing stress, anxiety, and depression and in dealing with many psychological problems. Exercise releases endorphins, which can improve your mood. Vigorous aerobic exercise can lower the level of pulse-quickening hormones released during stress and stimulate a feeling of well-being. Even a thirty-minute walk around the block can reduce anxiety. Try to schedule the exercise of your choice—running, swimming, walking—several times a week for at least forty-five minutes.

Exercise is one of the best ways to reduce stress. If the excess cortisol produced by stress is not burned up, there will be even more stress and overeating. Exercise also increases calorific expenditure and is an aid in weight reduction. Remember that weight can be a contributory factor to androgen problems. The higher the weight, the harder it is for a woman to ovulate. Finally, exercise will also relieve fluid retention and bloating associated with androgen excess.

Exercise is particularly recommended for diabetics because it increases metabolic rate, and diabetes is all about metabolism and how the body captures and uses energy.

STRESS MANAGEMENT

Stress occurs when there is an imbalance between the demands of your life and your ability to cope with those demands. Continued stress over a long period of time, for those with a heightened sensitivity to stress, will exhaust the adrenal glands, upset the balance of hormones, deplete the body's resources, and produce fatigue, changes in appetite, insomnia, depression, and problems such as androgen disorder. It can diminish the body's immune system, making you more vulnerable to disease. It may also bring on hypertension, a recognized factor in heart disease and some cancers.

Stress can kill.

We need a certain amount of challenge and stress in our life, but it should be a positive kind of stress, at a level that does not make us feel uncomfortable. It is negative stress, stress that is excessive and draining, that results in anxiety and eventual mental and physical breakdown. This is the kind of stress to avoid. If we cannot avoid it, we need to learn to deal with it in a positive way.

In the words of Joan Borysenko in *Minding the Body, Mending the Mind* (p. 16), it depends on our constitution: "Most of us will feel that life is out of control in some way. Whether we see this as a temporary situation whose resolution will add to our store of knowledge and experience, or as one more threat demonstrating life's dangers is the most crucial question both for the quality of our life and our physical health."

How Can I Reduce Stress?

Adrenal exhaustion and the accompanying overproduction of androgen hormone can be triggered by stress, so reducing stress is an important part of recovering from androgen disorder.

If stress levels are high in your life, stress reduction must be one of your first priorities. You don't need to take a month-long vacation to do this or change your life drastically. In addition to eating a healthy, balanced diet and exercising regularly (see previous sections in this chapter), the following recommendations will help you reduce the amount of stress in your life.

Sleep

Getting the right amount of sleep will significantly reduce the amount of stress in your life. If you wake up tired in the morning, you are not getting enough quality sleep.

Both lack of sleep and too much sleep will make you feel fatigued and stressed. Sleep is biologically necessary. Most of us need around eight hours a night, and if we do not get it we will not function well and it will affect our mood. Too much sleep can also get you out of condition, so you need to discover what is best for you. Sleep is vital for optimum brain power; without it we quickly become depressed, irritated, stressed, and fuzzy-headed. Eating, drinking alcohol, smoking, or exercising before bed can rob you of sleep. Studies have shown that to restore exhausted adrenals it is best to get to sleep before midnight.

Although no single prescription guarantees sweet sleep, lowering stress will enhance it. Learning how to relax will help you sleep better.

Relaxation

Many of us lead frantic, busy lives, and when we do finally get the time to relax we don't know how. We work hard, eat fast, play competitively, and toss and turn in our sleep. Our calendars are full, and we get tense if we don't achieve all that we think we should.

If stress reduction is your goal, it is essential that you relax and take time out. Relaxation is time for you. Each of us must find different ways to relax. Walking in the fresh air, for instance, watching a movie, reading a good book, seeing friends, drawing a picture, and playing an instrument are all ways to relax. Relaxation time is the time when you recharge the batteries and focus on what makes you feel good. Unfortunately, many women tend to neglect setting aside time and space for themselves. Many find it impossible to relax at all.

If you have problems relaxing, you need to learn how to take time out. One way to do this is to relax your whole body slowly, muscle by muscle. There are many tapes on the market that can help you through this process. Slowing down your breathing also gives you a chance to calm down.

Techniques like meditation and yoga can also have astonishing results on women who are stressed and tense. Try this simple routine: Choose a focus word or phrase—for example, "peace" or "happy." Sit quietly, and relax your body by tensing and then relaxing your muscles and breathing deeply. Say the focus word each time you exhale. If you lose concentration, simply return your thoughts to the word. Try this for just five minutes at first, and then gradually increase the amount of time. Do the routine at least once a day.

Imagery, a relaxation technique similar to daydreaming, involves allowing images to drift through your mind. Try to relax and let images come to you. Listen to tapes that invoke relaxation with the sounds of nature or someone describing the process of relaxation.

Such relaxation exercises done regularly can slow your breathing rate, calm your brain wave rhythms, and lower your blood pressure. Yoga also can relax tense muscles, teach you better breathing, lower your blood pressure, decrease your heart rate, and divert your mind from stress.

When you feel stressed, you could try counting to ten before you react or repeat to yourself some positive affirmation, such as "I am in control." Taking things a little more slowly than usual may also help beat stress. Soothing music can be beneficial, as can soaking in a hot tub, laughing more, interacting with others, cultivating outside interests, and diversions from your usual routine. There are so many delightful ways to relax. You should not think of it as time lost—it is time gained. When you return to your routine you will feel refreshed, energized, and in control and have a better perspective on things.

Relating to Others

With the disintegration of the community and family unit, lone-liness, isolation, and lack of intimacy is widespread. Partnership with people of both sexes, both sexual and nonsexual, is impor-tant for good health and stress reduction. Our lives find meaning not only through how we feel about ourselves but in our rela-tionships with others. All living beings need relationships with those of their own kind in order to be contented. No woman is an island. We need others to be happy, and we need many kinds of different relationships to feel fulfilled.

Researchers speculate that social ties might help us cope with stresses that lower our immunity. Immune cells have receptors that bind to stress hormones, and when this occurs the immune cells don't work as well and we are more likely to get ill.

One of the best ways you can reduce stress is by trying to build positive relationships with others. These relationships should not be ones that drain you but ones that make you feel good about yourself. If your friends are interested only in them-selves, or take you for granted, they are not friends. If you believe that friendship is all about your own needs being fulfilled, you are not a friend. Friendship is about giving and receiving and is based on the capacity to accept as well as to give love and respect. A good relationship with another person should add to your sense of zest and self-worth. If people sap your energy, you have been mixing with the wrong group of people.

Women who are happy in their relationships with others tend to be less stressed and anxious. On the other hand, some of us just naturally prefer solitude and find being around people stressful. If this is really the case, then it is better to stay solitary.

You have to find what makes you feel good. Just remember, though, that we develop as human beings through our emotional connections with others, and we continue to need relationships with others throughout our lives.

Laughter

One of the best ways to reduce stress is simply to try to have more fun with your life, to enjoy it. The positive emotions associated with laughter decrease stress hormones and increase the number of certain immune cells. Even if you are not the funny type, try seeing the lighter side of things and there will be positive benefits. If you are in a stressful situation, try to think of something light and amusing. You can deal with distress by using humor; laughter really can work wonders.

A recent study conducted in Sweden showed that those who went out to cultural events like shows at museums or even sports events tended to live longer than those who stayed at home. Increased social contact and reduced stress were the key factors here. Research also shows that music can reduce stress.

Faith

Having faith may also reduce stress. Researchers at Duke University Medical Center in Durham, North Carolina, recently found that people who attended religious services regularly had stronger immune systems. This might be due in part to the stress-reducing powers of social contact, but it is possible that prayer itself can relax us. It seems that turning to another source, or simply envisioning greater happiness for yourself, can make you feel more in control and less stressed.

Massage

In a study conducted by Dr. Gail Ironson, professor of psychology and psychiatry at the University of Miami in Coral Gables, she showed that massage is vital for a stronger immune system and reduced stress levels.

Massage relaxes your muscles and give you a much-needed time-out when you can revel in a feeling of being cared for.

A Positive Outlook

Having a positive outlook—seeing the glass as half full rather than half empty—can help you reduce the stress in your life. Trying to be more optimistic, instead of pessimistic, is a technique that can be learned. The next time you notice yourself reacting negatively to something, check yourself and see if you can this time see the positive side of things.

Helping Others

Focusing on the concerns of others can be a great stress reducer, as it takes our mind off our own worries. It can also counteract loneliness and depression.

The subject of stress management could fill a whole book. Only some of the many stress management techniques have been outlined above. Chapter 8 will explore other stress management techniques in more detail.

We turn now to caring for yourself as you learn to manage the symptoms of androgen disorder.

CARING FOR YOUR SKIN

The way skin looks is very important to the way we feel about ourselves, so we should take the best possible care of it we can.

Severe cases of acne require specialized medical care. Sometimes, though, treatment will not take effect for several months, and in the meantime there are ways you can help yourself.

Many believe that a greasy diet causes greasy skin, but so far it has not been proved that switching to a low-fat diet will cure acne. Acne is not caused by a poor diet, lack of sleep, or sex. Looking into these areas of your life, and trying to improve your diet or your sexual relationships, may make you feel better, but it won't make your acne go away.

There are four grades of acne, and you need to determine which one you have before you start treatment.

- Grade one: a few blackheads and whiteheads and possibly a few pimples.

- Grade two: whiteheads and blackheads with oily skin and pimples.

- Grade three: blackheads, whiteheads, pimples, and cysts that can appear on the face, shoulders, neck, and back.

- Grade four: large cysts that overlap each other and raised, thickened areas that can scar the skin.

For grade-one acne you can help yourself with frequent washing, which keeps the skin free of oil. Use a cloth to remove the outer layer of dead skin cells. Over-the-counter products are probably best. You should look for washes, gels, and creams that contain the chemical benzoyl peroxide. It starts with a concentration of 2.5 percent and goes up to 10 percent. It works to speed up oil secretions and skin cell turnover so that sebum is less likely to get trapped in the pores.

For grade-two acne your doctor can prescribe antibiotics either as a cream rubbed into the skin or in pill form. Tetracycline or erythromycin is usually the one prescribed. It is important that you take your antibiotic according to your doctor's instructions and don't stop midway; otherwise you may become immune to the antibiotic and it won't be as effective.

Because acne can have hormonal causes, many doctors are now prescribing a low-progesterone contraceptive pill to treat it.

For grade-three and grade-four acne, vitamin A treatments are available. Topical vitamin A derivatives are supplied as creams, gels, and lotions and work to dry up sebum. There are side effects, though: these include dry, inflamed skin and sensitivity to sunlight. Your doctor may prescribe oral vitamin A treatments. Vitamin A is a powerful anti-acne drug but can have dangerous side effects, including liver problems.

Acne and oily skin are such common problems that the number of products on the market for them is overwhelming. Here are a few tips:

- Heavy makeup can cause acne by blocking pores. Makeup should be kept to a minimum. Opaque foundations are the best to cover up acne. Cleanse thoroughly after you remove makeup. Never leave your makeup on at night. Choose oil-free moisturizers and makeup and use them in moderation. Opt for loose rather than pressed powders, which contain mineral oil, and powder blushes instead of creams. Look for the word *non-comedogenic* on labels.

- Always try to cleanse your skin at least twice a day.

- Don't pick or squeeze lesions—that can cause scarring.

- Choose oil-free sunscreens in gel or liquid form for your face, rather than a cream or a lotion.

- Avoid products that clog your pores. These include cold creams, products with mineral oils, and petroleum jelly.

- Some cosmetic companies, such as Clinique, Chanel, and Almay, make products especially for oily skin. Studies are inconclusive about whether the more expensive products are any better than the cheaper ones.

- Skin cleansers are readily available. They contain alcohol and dry the skin. They make you feel like your skin is cleaner because they have a slight sting, but their benefits are minimal.

- Soaps can be good cleansers, especially ones designed for oily skin. Choose a gentle soap or nonsoap cleanser.

- Abrasive scrubs are somewhat controversial. They do remove dead skin cells, but they can cause irritation and red skin. They dry out the skin and can actually make your sebum glands overproduce to compensate, which makes acne worse.

- Face packs remove oil temporally but do not help prevent or clear acne.

- When your acne eventually clears, and for most sufferers it eventually does, you'll most likely suffer from dry skin and need to use a moisturizer.

If traditional acne treatments seem too harsh, you might try the following recommendations:

- A study conducted by the Department of Dermatology of the Royal Prince Alfred Hospital in New South Wales, Australia, found that a 5 percent solution of tea tree oil was as effective as a 5 percent solution of benzoyl peroxide for most cases of acne and did not have the irritating side effects.

- Kombucha tea, which has antibacterial and immune-boosting qualities, has been found by many people to be beneficial to acne.

- Burdock root and red clover are powerful blood cleansers. Milk thistle aids the liver in cleansing the blood.

- A poultice made of chaparral, dandelion, and yellow dock root can be applied directly to the areas of the skin with acne.

- If your acne is severe, do not use steam treatments. They can make the condition worse. If the condition is mild to moderate, lavender, red clover, and strawberry leaves can be used as a steam sauna for the face.

- Some independent chemists sell a new product called Ketsugo, made from Isolutrol. Originally derived from shark's bile, this treatment is rich in antioxidants and can regulate sebum production and soften the skin.

- Other beneficial herbs include alfalfa, cayenne, dandelion root, and yellow dock root.

Although dietary changes cannot cure acne, certain food choices are beneficial:

- Eat a diet high in fiber to rid the body of toxins.

- Increase your intake of raw foods that contain oxalic acid, including almonds, beets, cashews, and Swiss chard. Exceptions include spinach and rhubarb; these contain oxalic acid but should be consumed in small amounts only.

- Eat more foods rich in zinc, including shellfish, soybeans, sunflower seeds, and a small amount of raw nuts. Zinc is an antibacterial agent and a necessary element in the oil-producing glands of the skin. A diet low in zinc may promote flare-ups.

- Ensure an adequate intake of B vitamins, which are important for healthy skin tone.

- Flaxseed oil and primrose oil are good sources of essential fatty acids needed to keep skin smooth and clear and to repair damaged skin cells.

- Avoid alcohol, sugar, processed food, iodized salt, fish, kelp, onions, butter, caffeine, cheese, chocolate, eggs, fish, fried foods, spicy foods, margarine, meat, poultry, wheat, soft drinks, and foods containing brominated vegetable oils.

CARING FOR YOUR HAIR

The hair shaft is covered in tightly overlapping cuticle cells and a thin coating of oil.

Teasing, blow drying, dyes, and permanents separate the layers of the cuticle cells, causing split ends, or at the very least swell the cells, making the hair surface uneven. The smoother the surface of the hair, the shinier it will be, which is why damaged hair looks dull and dry. Conditioners can smooth out the cuticle cells and coat the hair with oil to make it shine again, but they are only a temporary solution.

If your hair is not dry and thin but oily, frequent washing with mild shampoo will temporarily make it look better.

Removing Unwanted Hair

Many women remove hair from their legs and underarms to fit our culture's definition of femininity. For those of us with normal hair growth, the following methods are effective and all that is needed. But for women with androgen disorder, the usual methods yield poor results. If you are spending too much time plucking, shaving, and waxing, it is time to seek advice from a doctor.

Plucking

A popular method of hair removal—especially on the face—plucking can cause injury to the skin when the hair is pulled out of the root. Infection is also a possibility.

Waxing

Just like plucking, waxing pulls the hair out by the root. It is usually done by a beautician. The skin looks very smooth afterward, and hair takes time to grow back unless you have an androgen excess problem, in which case you will need to wax again in a few days.

Creams

Known as depilatories, these creams dissolve hair. They can cause skin irritation and redness if left on too long, but they do not work if left on for too short a time. If you find the amount of time that is right for you, using these creams is better than plucking and waxing, but it is still not a long-term solution.

Razors

Because shaving your face seems such a masculine thing to do, many women don't like doing it, but it is in fact one of the best short-term solutions. It will not, as everyone seems to believe, make the hair grow back thicker and faster. It only feels thicker because you have cut the hair off at the root, where it was thicker anyway.

If you use a good razor, shaving is not harmful to the skin. It is important to wet the hair for several minutes before shaving and to use a shaving cream. Moisturizer should be used after shaving.

Electrolysis

Electrolysis destroys the hair follicle with heat or electricity. Proper electrolysis requires great skill, and even then it does not work for all women. It can be painful, and it can also mark the skin and cause inflammation. It will destroy the hair follicle so hair won't grow back, but other follicles then become active, and it is hard for electrolysis to keep up. The process is very slow and also very costly. It is best to use this method as a supplement to hormonal therapy.

If you want to have electrolysis done, be sure to choose a skilled electrologist who uses disposable needles.

Hair Loss

Androgen-related hair loss needs to be treated by a doctor, but you can help yourself by getting all your nutrients, exercising regularly, and decreasing the amount of stress in your life.

Eat plenty of foods rich in biotin and use hair-care products containing biotin, which is needed for healthy hair and skin. Good food sources include brewer's yeast, brown rice, green peas, lentils, oats, soybeans, sunflower seeds, and walnuts. Ensure an adequate intake of B vitamins, vitamin C, vitamin E, and zinc, all of which improve the health and growth of hair.

Avoid products that are not natural on the hair, and avoid rough treatment to the hair. Do not use a fine-toothed comb or towel-dry your hair. Also, do not use a blow dryer or other heated appliances on your hair; let it dry naturally. Do not comb your hair until it is dry, as wet hair tends to break off.

Remember that it is normal to lose around a hundred hairs a day. If you think you are losing more than this, see a doctor.

NATURAL PROGESTERONE

The great majority of women with androgen disorder and anovulation are progesterone deficient. If you do not ovulate, progesterone is not secreted by the ovary in sufficient quantities to counteract the effects of estrogen.

Many women feel uncomfortable, nauseated, and irritable when they take the synthetically manufactured drug progestin, so an alternative to consider is a natural progesterone cream. Progesterone cream balances estrogen dominance symptoms such as low sex drive, fatigue, water retention, bone loss, weight gain, and low adrenal function.

The progesterone in skin cream is absorbed into the fatty layer beneath your skin; from there, it travels to the bloodstream. Sometimes it may take several weeks for you to feel any benefits. It is important *not* to use more of the cream in an attempt to speed results.

There are many progesterone creams available, and you need to exercise caution when you select one. The one most highly recommended by natural therapists and by Gittleman (*Before the*

Change) is Pro-Gest from Professional and Technical Services. It can be ordered from Uni Key Health Systems (see Resources section) if you can't find it in a health-food store. You may also prefer to take natural progesterone as an oral capsule.

MEASURING HORMONE LEVELS

Home ovulation kits can tell you if you are ovulating or not. You can buy these at your local supermarket or drugstore. However, if you want to know for sure if you have an androgen imbalance, ovulation testing is not enough: you need to have your hormone levels measured. Until recently, you could be tested for levels of estrogen, progesterone, and testosterone only by blood and urine tests. In most cases this would involve a visit to your doctor. Now, however, a new method, the saliva test has become available. It is cheaper and easier to administer, and you don't have to visit a doctor to take it—you can do it yourself at home.

If your doctor thinks you should take a saliva test, you will be given instructions, sample collection materials, and mailing instructions to send the test to a lab. If you don't want to visit your doctor, you can order saliva tests for up to four hormones from Aeron Life Cycles in California. Aeron will provide you with materials for saliva collection and mailing. The cost is around fifty dollars per test, and you can usually get results back within ten days. Aeron makes it clear that its direct-to-consumer tests are meant only to monitor changes in hormonal levels. Remember that your hormone levels fluctuate on a daily basis. So bear in mind that a test on one day may differ from one taken a few days before. Also, the results will be affected by the day of your menstrual cycle—remember that androgen levels peak at ovulation. If you find the test results hard to interpret, the best thing to do is to see a health care provider. For more information on measuring hormone levels, see chapter 7.

Taking a saliva test is easy, convenient, and private. Hormones remain stable at room temperature, so they can be stored easily before you send them to the lab by mail. Be careful that you have no bleeding or infections in your gums, as this could affect the test results. When you take the test, chew some gum to generate saliva, take note of the date and time of day, and spit into the tube provided before sealing it.

EVERY WOMAN IS UNIQUE

The advice given in this chapter is based on research on and case histories of women who suffer from hormonal imbalance and what worked for them. It is important to remember, though, that each one of you is unique. Just as a normal androgen level for one woman may be abnormal for another, the same applies to self-help and preventive measures. What works for someone else may not work for you. We all have different hormone levels, different metabolic rates, different bodies, and different personalities. You need to find what works for you.

Though self-help techniques such as diet and exercise are beneficial in the management of androgen disorder, they are not front-line treatments. Many of you may prefer to see a doctor or endocrinologist. Normally the kind of self-help techniques recommended here will be the same as those offered by an alternative medicine practitioner. However, should you be diagnosed with androgen disorder, the first person you will usually see will not be an alternative practitioner but a doctor or endocrinologist who specializes in hormonal problems. The following chapter will explain what he or she is likely to say and do and what kind of treatment will be offered.

7

Conventional Treatment and Procedures

Without a doubt, androgen disorder can destroy the quality of your life. Hair loss is humiliating. Facial and body hair growth is embarrassing. Acne is irritating. Irregular periods make you feel uncomfortable. Weight gain and fatigue slow you down.

Anything that destroys the quality of your life deserves medical attention. It is a shame that misinformation about hormones and how to treat hormonal problems prevents many women with health problems from seeking treatment. Hormones are not as incomprehensible, mysterious, and erratic as many of us have been led to believe, and treatment, if properly administered, is safe and effective.

For many women the first step is a change in attitude. Perhaps you have a cluster of the symptoms associated with androgen disorder. If this is the case, you need to admit that you have a significant health problem. This is never easy. We all like to think we are invulnerable, and ignoring symptoms can easily become a way of life.

The following ten points reinforce just how potentially serious the condition can be and how important it is that you not ignore your symptoms and that you seek medical advice:

1. If you have androgen disorder, the balance of hormones in your body has been upset. Basically, your body is in a state of crisis. Your body was not designed to lose hair, have male hair growth patterns, have acne, and not menstruate. The endocrine system revolves around a complex system of checks, balances, and interrelationships. Problems with one gland are eventually going to affect other glands and then affect your whole body. Poor health will result.

2. There is a strong possibility that you are insulin-resistant; you may even be diabetic.

3. You could be suffering from some underlying disease that needs immediate treatment.

4. You may be at increased risk of heart disease.

5. If you have an androgen disorder, you are in danger of developing cancer of the womb.

6. You could be more likely to develop ovarian cancer.

7. An androgen disorder might make you infertile. The longer the condition goes untreated, the greater the chance that the infertility will not reverse itself.

8. Symptoms are easier to treat when they are mild. Don't wait until symptoms get severe before you see a doctor.

9. Hirsutism is a problem that often won't just go away. No amount of plucking, shaving, waxing, or applying creams is going to really help.

10. The symptoms of androgen disorder can destroy the quality of your life.

DIAGNOSIS

The first thing your doctor will do is ask you a series of questions about your symptoms, health, and lifestyle. Should you have irregular periods, an ultrasound will screen for abnormalities.

Should you have classic hirsute symptoms, you'll be asked about their history and development. Whether the condition developed rapidly or slowly gives an indication of the seriousness of the situation. Has the hirsutism come on quickly, or been progressive for several years? Has virilization occurred? Has hair growth changed or remained the same? Do you have a family history of infertility and hirsutism? Have there been disturbances in your menstrual cycle? Has your voice deepened? Has your libido decreased? Have you lost hair? Gained or lost weight? What about fatigue, skin changes? How much do you exercise? Have you taken androgenic medications or steroids?

A physical examination may then follow. The type and pattern of hair growth and acne will be noted. The presence of virilization, leakage from the breasts, and other abnormalities will be detected. It is important at this stage to determine if hirsutism is really present.

If your symptoms suggest hormonal problems, your doctor will want to confirm this with tests. These tests may be carried out by a hospital, by an endocrinologist, or by your doctor. The tests and screening will determine what your androgen levels are and whether the problem is ovarian, adrenal, or both.

Testing Hormone Levels

There are two methods of measuring your level of testosterone. The most commonly used is the blood test. It is important that you have a blood test that measures levels of both bound and free testosterone. Free testosterone affects the body more quickly, but bound testosterone gradually converts to free testosterone, so if either form of testosterone is elevated it is significant. A test of testosterone levels only will also not be sufficient. Remember that the other androgens act as sources to make more testosterone, so their levels need to be monitored too.

The problem with the blood test is that it may not always be accurate, for a number of reasons. First, different labs have different methods of measurement, and some are more accurate and dependable than others. Second, your androgen levels will fluctuate. A test on one day may yield different results than a test on another day. The time of day the test was taken, as well as where you are in your menstrual cycle, is also significant. Third, androgen levels fluctuate with age. They are at their highest in the late teens and early twenties and gradually decline after that. Finally, some women with normal androgen levels may be manifesting symptoms of androgen disorder such as acne or hair growth. The problem in these cases is the response of a woman's skin or hair to testosterone, which can't be measured by a blood test.

Understanding blood test lab results is not always easy. The best thing to do if you are confused is to look at the normal range printed on the lab chart and see where you are. Remember, though, that these are averages and they do not fit all situations. Sometimes labs set the normal level a little too high. According to Dr. Geoffrey Redmond (*Women's Hormones*, p. 37), "The average testosterone level in a woman is about 40ng/dl in comparison to 400ng/dl or higher for a man. A high level for a woman would be 120ng/dl . . . but women who have levels of 50ng/dl often notice androgen changes on their skin and hair."

If levels are dangerously high, say 150ng/dl, your condition is very serious. You will need urgent treatment. You could have a serious disease or adrenal and ovarian tumors. You should be tested for congenital adrenal hyperplasia as well as thyroid problems and Cushing's syndrome.

You can also have your testosterone levels checked by a saliva test. The saliva test is cheaper and easier to administer than other types of tests, but it measures only your level of free testosterone.

Only a small percentage of androgen is in a free, biologically active form. With androgen disorder it is important to know levels of both free and bound testosterone. According to Dr. James Dabbs, a professor and researcher in the department of psychology at Georgia State University in Atlanta, salivary measurements of testosterone are compounded by the same complex problems that plague blood tests. However, the advantage of a saliva test is that you can do it in the privacy of your own home.

Although both blood and saliva tests have their uncertainties and can never be entirely accurate for each woman's individual circumstances, they can be very useful indeed. Not only can they let you know immediately if there is a problem with your androgen levels, but they also provide a way for you to monitor your hormone levels over time.

Your doctor may also want to run a dexamethasone suppression test. This is a very useful test that tries to determine how much of a woman's androgens are coming from her adrenals and how much of them are coming from her ovaries. This test may take several days and involves the administration of the drug dexamethasone. Sometimes it is the only way to determine if androgen is coming from the adrenals.

If all the tests show that your androgen levels are normal and you still have androgen-related problems such as acne or thinning hair, the problem may well be the sensitivity of your skin to normal levels of androgen. This can be diagnosed and treated with androgen antagonists, discussed later.

TREATING ANDROGEN DISORDER

Being diagnosed with androgen disorder can lead to feelings of anger, confusion, and guilt. But this is often because of ignorance about the condition. It may take time to come to terms with your condition, and you may be fearful about what it all means. These fears usually disperse once you become more familiar with the condition. One thing you should realize, however, is that most doctors believe that you can never fully correct androgen disorder. It is a condition that will need continuous treatment, until the ovaries finally stop making androgen at menopause.

Treatment will suppress symptoms, but symptoms will return in most cases if treatment stops. For instance, even after hormonal treatment has restored fertility and a woman has a baby, if the treatment is not continued postpartum, androgen imbalance will probably return.

Because of the complexity of the androgenic system and because each woman's body is different, treatments vary according to each patient's individual circumstances. Treatment, however, when safely administered, is very often beneficial and effective.

Should you be diagnosed with androgen disorder your doctor will want to determine whether you wish to be treated for fertility problems, hirsutism, irregular menses, or any other androgen related disorder. You will be given a pregnancy test, because treatment of hirsutism is contraindicated for pregnant women. If your blood glucose levels are high, you will immediately be given tablets to lower your blood pressure. These are called *hypoglycemic drugs*— or drugs to stimulate insulin production. Should you be overweight, diet changes and exercise will be recommended. They are especially beneficial not only for people with androgen disorders but also for those with diabetes, elevated cholesterol, and high blood pressure. It is not wise, however, to delay seeking treatment until you lose weight. Loosing weight is hard and may take time. The sooner you get treatment for androgen disorder, the better, because symptoms have a tendency to get more severe the older you get.

Once it has been discovered that there is androgen excess, in order for successful treatment to begin, it is first important to establish the goals of therapy. This involves deciding if you wish to become pregnant in the near future. Many hormonal treatments cannot be pursued if you are pregnant, so deciding whether or not to seek fertility treatment is the first step.

The Pill

If you do not wish to become pregnant, the usual treatment for androgen excess, whether hirsutism and other symptoms are present or not, is the oral contraceptive pill. According to Dr. James Douglas, "It is in the best interests of women with irregular periods due to PCO to go on the Pill to lower their risk of heart disease and cancer."

The Pill suppresses the secretion of the reproductive hormones and decreases ovarian androgen production. Doctors don't quite know why, but the Pill also decreases adrenal androgen production. The progesterone in the Pill works on androgen receptors, and the estrogen in the Pill decreases levels of free testosterone in the blood. The Pill should be taken on a daily basis on a four-week schedule. It is important to monitor androgen levels regularly to ensure that things are returning to normal.

Sometimes, though, the Pill can make things worse if it is too high in estrogen and you are already suffering from symptoms of estrogen dominance. Make sure you test not just your androgen levels but also your estrogen and progesterone levels to determine the correct hormonal dosage of the Pill you will be prescribed.

Suppression of Ovarian Androgen

The Pill prevents reproductive hormones from being released by the pituitary gland. Ovulation and hormonal secretion from the ovaries does not occur. Estrogen, progesterone, and androgen levels decrease, but because the Pill contains estrogen and progesterone, the decrease in these hormones goes unnoticed.

Sometimes the decrease in androgen is not enough and other medications will be needed, but for most women with androgen disorders the Pill is the best remedy. It lowers androgens and regulates bleeding. It can have unpleasant side effects, though, and these include nausea, weight gain, dizziness, and fatigue.

Suppression of Adrenal Androgen

If your androgen disorder is caused by overproduction of androgens by the adrenal gland, then the most effective form of treatment that suppresses the production of androgens from the adrenal gland is small doses of the drug glucorticoid. Prednisone and dexamethasone (decadron) are also used. They can be effective, but only if the androgens are coming from the adrenal gland. If the dosage is correct, the adrenal gland will still be able to secrete cortisol.

GnRH Analogues

Some women cannot take the Pill, so the next resort is GnRH analogues. A GnRH analogue stimulates the pituitary and estrogen levels go up. When the pituitary stops stimulating the ovary, estrogen and androgen secretion stop. The endometrium will now shed. If GnRH is continued, estrogen and androgen levels continue to fall. Estrogen replacement therapy can be given to limit the side effects of estrogen deficiency, such as hot flashes.

GnRH analogues are rather cumbersome, as they suppress all the hormones coming from the ovary, which (apart from androgen) then need to be replaced by other drugs. GnRH analogues are also expensive, and they should be considered a last resort.

Hormonal Therapy for Irregular Periods

If you don't want to go on the Pill, don't want to get pregnant, and have no other symptoms apart from irregular menses, you will be given monthly progesterone and/or estrogen-related therapy. This will induce a monthly bleed and prevent the continued estrogen stimulation of the endometrium, which carries with it a high risk of cancer, as well as protecting against health risks associated with amenorrhea, such as osteoporosis.

Treatment for Hirsutism, Alopecia, and Acne

If hirsutism or alopecia are present, treatment should be undertaken immediately, because these conditions tend to be progressive. Hormonal therapy may sometimes take several months to have a noticeable effect. Also, in most cases the problem will never completely go away, but it will be significantly alleviated.

Hormonal therapy for hirsutism attempts to stop new terminal hair from growing. It may also thin out terminal hairs already present and limit their further growth. It cannot reverse the androgen-induced transformation of vellus to terminal hair that has already occurred. In some instances, hormonal therapy may take up to a year to be effective, so mechanical means of hair removal can be used in the meantime.

Androgen Antagonists

The treatments discussed so far are hormonal therapies designed to lower the amount of androgens in your body; this type of treatment is called *suppression*. Another set of treatments can block the effect of androgens on skin and hair. This type of treatment is called *anti-androgen* or *androgen antagonist treatment*. Antagonists make the oil gland or hair follicle less receptive to androgen stimulation. They cannot be 100 percent effective, though; sometimes the problem remains but in a milder form.

Anti-androgens are most effective for women who have normal levels of androgens but whose skin or hair is very sensitive to the effects of androgens. In general, androgen skin problems respond best to anti-androgens. Anti-androgens tend to work well when testosterone levels are low, so they are often used in combination with other medications that lower hormone levels.

Anti-androgens take time to work. Acne improves within a few weeks or months, but unwanted hair growth or baldness takes much longer, sometimes several years, to improve. There is reason to be concerned about possible birth defects if you take an anti-androgen during pregnancy. A highly reliable form of contraception must be taken if you are to be put on anti-androgen therapy.

If you are considering anti-androgens therapy, you should delay pregnancy for a year or two. Whether or not you choose to do this is an individual decision. It depends on what is more important to you: getting rid of the effects of hirsutism and delaying childbirth or trying to conceive now. If you have hirsutism and PCO, you will need hormonal treatment to ovulate and get pregnant.

None of the anti-androgen drugs mentioned here are officially labeled for use with androgen disorder or have FDA (Food and Drug Administration) approval. In all cases, the drugs were developed to treat other conditions. Concern about side effects, birth defects, and the huge cost of obtaining FDA approval are among the reasons for this, but it also shows that one of the most common female hormone problems is still not being taken seriously as a medical condition that needs drugs developed specifically for it.

The treatment most often used in the United States is SPA (Spironolactone). It was introduced thirty years ago to block the hormone aldosterone, but it also blocks testosterone and other androgens by antagonizing the androgen receptors and suppressing various enzymes involved in androgen production. The drug has a high success rate, but it will not work for all women, and additional drugs may be needed. There may be side effects when treatment starts, including frequent urination, dizziness, fatigue, headaches, and frequent menstrual bleeding.

SPA is one of the most effective treatments for hirsutism. Since it acts differently from the Pill, it is possible to combine the two in treatment. The use of SPA together with the Pill will eliminates the problem of irregular periods associated with SPA and also provides contraception.

Dexamethasone or prednisone can be used to treat hirsutism. Oral estrogen may also be used for those who can't tolerate the Pill. Oral estrogen antagonizes the effect of androgens at the hair follicle level. High doses of progesterone also decrease testosterone levels. However, the side effects may be unpleasant and will include depression, hot flashes, liver problems, and irregular bleeding.

Cyproterone acetate (CPA) is a strong progesterone and anti-androgen. Developed as a treatment for cancer, it also decreases testosterone levels and antagonizes the effects of androgens. It acts as an effective birth control pill, too. Side effects include bloating and depression and may include adrenal problems and loss of libido. This drug does not have FDA approval and is not yet available in the United States.

Cimetidine (brand name Tagamet) may also be an anti-androgen. It blocks the release of acid to help reduce stomach irritation, but at the same time it has some blocking effect on androgen receptors. Recent studies show that it is not really an effective treatment for hirsutism.

Flutamide (Eulexin) is a new drug. Developed a few years ago specifically as an anti-androgen, it is effective in treating hirsutism. Its official labeling is, however, as a treatment for prostate cancer. The drug seems to be effective, but it has some side effects. The biggest danger is liver disease. It is very expensive and therefore is not often used when treating androgen disorders.

Ketoconazole (Nizoral) is an antifungal antibiotic that has been found to be an anti-antagonist. It is seldom used, though, because it carries with it a serious risk of liver damage. It is available in skin cream form, used to try to block androgens in the skin.

Finasteride (Proscar) is a new drug introduced to relieve prostate problems. It prevents DHT from converting to testosterone, so there is the as yet uninvestigated possibility that it can help with hirsutism and alopecia.

Ovulation Induction

If you are not ovulating and want to have a baby, you should begin ovulation induction.

Hirsutism, acne, and alopecia cannot be treated while fertility is being pursued, because the treatment would increase the risk of birth defects. Also, ovulation restoration does not lower androgen levels enough to be therapeutic for hirsutism. So although you may ovulate, your hirsutism is unlikely to improve.

If your weight is high, the first recommendation is to lose weight. Obesity is a contributory factor in anovulation. The next step is to take the fertility drug clomiphene citrate, known as clomid. Your body must be able to produce estrogen for this to work. If you bleed after being withdrawn from a course of progesterone pills, clomid will be given. If you don't bleed, it is probable that your estrogen levels are dangerously low and estrogen-related therapy will be needed. Screening for early menopause should also take place.

After a period, which may need to be induced by taking progesterone, clomid pills are taken orally for a period of about five days. The first dose is usually 50mg a day and is taken between days three to five in a menstrual cycle. Clomid increases the secretion of reproductive hormones from the pituitary, and a dominant follicle grows. Ovulation usually occurs within seven days after taking the last clomid pill. Ovulation is confirmed by temperature tests and ultrasound. If ovulation does not occur, clomid dosage is increased to 100mg a day and then to 150mg until the 250mg limit is reached. Sometimes at around 200mg dexamethasone is given to decrease adrenal androgen and to increase sensitivity to clomid. Clomid therapy is usually given for around six months. It works for about 60 percent of women, and chances of getting pregnant while on clomid are around 40 percent. The chances of multiple pregnancy and miscarriage are slight. Side effects include hot flashes, vaginal dryness, and headaches.

If follicles mature but fail to ovulate while you are on clomid, you'll be given a shot of human chorionic gonadotropin when the follicle reaches 18mm to induce ovulation. If clomid does not work for you, stronger fertility treatments will be needed.

Pergonal may now be used to stimulate ovulation, and it has a very high success rate. It is mainly used for women with low levels of hormones to stimulate the ovaries and estrogen. Pergonal will make your ovaries release several eggs, because it contains human chorionic gonadotrophin, which stimulates the ovaries.

Fertility treatments are improving all the time, and a number of other amazing drugs are available for women as well as clomid and pergonal. There may be unpredictable side effects such as depression, pain from overstimulated ovaries, insomnia, nausea, and hot flashes. Also, the risk of multiple births is higher while on medication. The symptoms are not usually serious, though, and if fertility drugs make your periods come back or help you conceive, they are well worth taking.

Nonhormonal Treatments Recommended by Doctors

Retinoids

Retinoids are a form of Vitamin A. They dry the skin and makes it less oily. They are available in skin cream form as Tretinoin (Retin A) and as a pill, Isotretinoin (Accutane). Side effects of retinoids include drying of the skin and possible irritation. Accutane is more effective than Tretinoin, but it can cause serious birth defects.

Antibiotics

Antibiotics have been used to treat acne for many years. They work on infections that cause acne and they prevent the growth of bacteria. Tetracycline, minocycine, erythromycin, and trimethroprimsulfa are most often used. Tetracycline is the most cost-efficient, although it is not as effective as the more expensive minocycline. Side effects of tetracycline include yeast infection. If this is a problem, perhaps erythromycin may work, but it can upset the stomach. This drug is also dangerous in combination with other medications, so always check with your doctor for safety. Antibiotics may cause contraceptives to be less effective.

Antibiotics are available as skin creams such as benzoyl peroxide. Oxy 5 and Oxy 10 (Smithkline Beecham) are also available. Sometimes these creams can make the face become red and sore.

Surgery

Until the 1960s, surgery was the most common form of treatment for PCO. A deep wedge of tissue containing the extra cells in the ovary was removed by surgery. The improvement, however, tended to be short term.

This operation, called *bilateral ovarian wedge resection,* was successful in some instances. Risks include adhesions in the pelvis and fertility problems. Today, surgery is considered far too drastic a solution and hormonal therapy is preferred.

If a tumor is present in the ovaries, however, surgery may be the only option. If you have surgery, it is essential that you get counseling and support.

Treating Precocious Puberty

In cases of precocious puberty, doctors will examine the brain with X-rays or other techniques to produce images of the brain. If there is a tumor causing the disorder, it will show up in these tests. Blood tests will also be run to rule out thyroid problems or tumors elsewhere in the body. Urinary and blood plasma analysis for androgen steroids and cortisol will determine if there are congenital adrenal problems or Cushing's syndrome. Plasma testosterone will be checked to see if there are tumors in the testes or ovaries.

The condition can be treated with progesterone acetate or GnRH analogues. These drugs will inhibit ovary-stimulating hormones or the pituitary's response to them. If progesterone is used, bone maturation does not cease, but menstruation and breast development stop. Bones will continue to grow and may stop prematurely. GnRH analogues, however, act upon the pituitary gland to return it completely to a prepuberty state, except for pubic hair that has grown, which will not go away. Reassurance and psychological counseling for both parents and the child will be needed, because precocity is an upsetting experience for all concerned.

If there is an underlying physical defect, treatment involves correcting that. Tumors may be surgically removed.

Treating Delayed Puberty

In cases of delayed puberty, blood tests will be taken to measure the levels of sex hormones, thyroid hormone, and cortisol. If hypothalamic or pituitary disease is suspected, a CAT scan will be done to check for tumors or defects.

If all hormonal tests have normal results, puberty will be induced with low doses of sex hormones. Treatment usually begins between the ages of fifteen and sixteen. Once menstruation occurs, hormonal treatment is reduced to a minimum.

Treating Androgen Deficiency at Menopause

To relieve the uncomfortable physical and emotional symptoms of menopause and decrease the risk of heart disease and osteoporosis, many women are placed on estrogen replacement therapy at menopause. It is still not standard, however, to place menopausal women on androgen as well as estrogen replacement therapy, even though androgen deficiency at menopause can cause loss of sex drive and energy, as well as depression.

Many women who have taken androgen replacement at menopause do report feeling much better, and there is growing evidence that it is beneficial.

According to Dr. Susan Rako, "The unique role of supplemental testosterone for maintaining vital and sexual energy must challenge the automatic assumption that hormone replacement therapy means estrogen and progesterone. For many women HRT means estrogen, progesterone and testosterone" (*Hormone of Desire*, p. 94).

Not all doctors, however, are as enthusiastic as Rako. Although many admit that the addition of testosterone to HRT may make some women feel better, many doctors, such as Redmond (*Women's Hormones*, p. 468) express "great concern" about androgen therapy at menopause and its side effects. Other doctors, such as Dr. James Douglas, prescribe it according to individual need:

"It is still not usual to use male and female hormone replacement at menopause. I have found that some feel better when they are given it. I prescribe it according to individual need. If a woman says she feels lethargic and has no energy, she might benefit from androgen therapy. I warn her of the risks." Although the libido tends to improve on androgen therapy, there is a downside. Levels of good cholesterol decrease, heart disease is more likely, and there may be an increase in androgenic symptoms such as hair loss, hair in unwanted places, and increased skin oiliness and acne. These symptoms can be avoided if the testosterone dosage is low.

The key factor here is determining the level of testosterone replacement that is right for you. Most of us need only very small amounts of testosterone to feel better. Until recently, the only testosterone replacement therapy that was available was far more potent than necessary. Estratest has been the leading pharmaceutical used to treat testosterone deficiency in women. Even in low dosages it still contains too much testosterone, and this has been shown to place a strain on liver function. Many women who have been placed on Estratest have felt worse, not better.

Now, however, there are forms of testosterone therapy that are milder and made in a micronized form. Testosterone can be made in a wide variety of other forms: skin creams, skin gel, tablets, and vaginal suppositories. These forms can produce amazing results, but doctors are still looking for the right way to administer testosterone and for the right dose.

If your testosterone levels fall below 20ng/dl, you might want to consider testosterone therapy. You will have to weigh the potential benefits of testosterone therapy against possible future side effects. The optimal level for energy and libido is between 30 and 60ng/dl. Levels can usually be determined by a blood test, so if you feel loss of energy and lack of interest in sex, it is worth having your androgen levels checked. If they are low, then you need to discuss with your doctor the option of androgen replacement.

Should you decide to go ahead with testosterone therapy, you need to make sure that you are given a dose that is correct for your needs. Remember that every body is different. You need to find the level of testosterone replacement that is unique to you. Regular blood tests can determine this. You and your doctor need to work together to find out what is most suitable.

If your life circumstances are stressful, of course no amount of testosterone replacement at menopause is going to change things. Testosterone is not a magic wand that will give you fantastic sexual vigor and energy. If levels are adequate, however, it can help you enjoy the level of sexuality that is natural to you and feel better equipped to deal with life's ups and downs.

Hormonal therapy for androgen disorder may not suit everyone, but it tends to be very effective. Acne clears, skin tone improves, hair growth and loss often corrects itself, and infertility reverses itself.

If you do decide to have treatment, it is vital to take the trouble to find a doctor who is going to work with you and really consider your individual circumstances. Many women complain that their doctor never listens and never has enough time for them. Many of us leave the office with unanswered questions, costly prescriptions, and inconvenient follow-up appointments. The problem is caused by busy doctors and reticent patients; we often feel intimidated and embarrassed to talk about our problems. If you are really dissatisfied, change to another doctor, but you might benefit from getting the most out of the time you spend with your doctor. Make sure you write down everything you want to know and talk about. Be organized, and tactfully interrupt if you feel your doctor isn't listening to your concerns. Speak up for yourself. Remember that you have a right to be there.

Your doctor is there to help you. Make sure he or she takes your concerns seriously. Remind yourself that androgen disorders are a medical condition that can have severe health risks if left untreated. Remind yourself that you deserve to feel as healthy as you possibly can.

8

Alternative Therapies

Although a change in diet and lifestyle may be all that is needed to banish androgen disorder for a few women, the great majority need extra help to keep their androgen levels stable and will begin a program of hormonal therapy prescribed by a doctor. Should this be the case for you, you may want to complement your conventional treatment or find something to help it work more effectively.

If this is you, then you join the thousands of people around the world who turn to alternative therapies for virtually every health complaint. In the last ten years or so, alternative health care has enjoyed tremendous growth, and there are now many treatment options available to the consumer. Also, the divide that used to exist between the alternative and the orthodox approach is no longer as wide, and learning and interaction is taking place between the two to offer the best health care treatment available.

What we consider alternative health care has always existed; it is as old as humankind. For centuries, people have turned to the healing power of touch, to special diets, to herbal remedies, to hot and cold water to stimulate circulation, or to manipulating the body's energy fields to promote health and well-being. Orthodox medicine does not have such a long history to support its use; it did not begin to develop until the late nineteenth century. Often considered the medicine of the West, orthodox medicine stresses the importance of cure, of finding a drug to kill a disease or to correct a chemical imbalance in the body. Doctors tend to be impersonal in their search for a quick answer to the problem and the belief that it can be fixed by medication. The problem, though, is that often in destroying what is harmful, drugs also destroy what is beneficial. Antibiotics are a case in point. They kill harmful bacteria that cause infection, but at the same time they destroy the body's beneficial bacteria. Many drugs can also have unpleasant and dangerous side effects. Yet despite this, there is much that is good about the orthodox approach. It often is a lifesaver. It comes to its own in times of crisis, and millions of lives have been saved by it, where alternative medicine might have failed.

Ideally, conventional and alternative medicine can overlap and the patient can benefit from both.

If you are considering an alternative treatment, it is advisable to see an orthodox doctor first to check that no underlying disease is at work. After consulting with your doctor, you may wish to investigate alternative therapies to complement medication given by your doctor. Always check with your doctor to ensure that what you are taking is safe, though.

Alternative medicine can be very beneficial for those who need to reduce stress levels and make lifestyle and diet changes. A natural healer, rather than an orthodox doctor, will sometimes be better qualified to look at your whole lifestyle, physical and emotional, determine where there is an imbalance, and show you how you can become actively involved in your own recovery.

If you decide to seek help from alternative medicine, the sheer number of different therapies available can be overwhelming. From acupuncture to macrobiotics and meditation to hypnotherapy and yoga, many therapies offer treatments for hormonal problems in women.

Which one to chose? Which one works best? Unfortunately, there is no definitive answer. Different therapies work for different women. It would be wise to read about the various options available, so that you understand the principles behind them before you go for a consultation. Some will appeal to you more than others. If you are going for a consultation, make sure you check out the experience, qualifications, and background of the practitioner you visit. There are a lot of charlatans out there trying to cash in on people's vulnerability and on the current popularity of alternative therapy.

In practice, natural therapies can be divided into two categories: psychological therapies, which retrain the mind and emotions into healthier patterns, and therapies that begin with the body and affect both physical and psychological states. Improving your mental state often improves your overall health, and by the same token improving your physical health often has a positive effect on your mind. Many alternative therapies treat both mind and body at the same time. Naturopathy and Yoga, for example, address both physical and psychological states.

This dual approach can have many benefits for sufferers of androgen disorder. For example, psychological therapy such as hypnosis can help sufferers reduce stress in their lives or see themselves in a more positive light. Meanwhile, a more physical approach like acupuncture can alleviate symptoms and help to create physiological changes such as a reduction in blood sugar levels and improved circulation.

NATUROPATHY

We begin with naturopathy because it can be an amalgam of physical and psychological therapies. The term originated in the late nineteenth century, but it can be traced back thousands of years.

People have always believed that healing will occur naturally in the human body, if it is given what it truly needs: clean water, a balanced diet, fresh air, sunlight, exercise, and adequate sleep. Rather than finding disease and killing it, the body is helped to establish its own state of good health with various recommendations and techniques. The emphasis is on prevention rather than cure, and the body is strengthened to fight disease. The naturopath's code can therefore be summed up by one simple statement: the body is self-healing. The body strives toward health and has the power to heal itself. We can see this ourselves when a scar forms over a wound or our body temperature adjusts naturally or our immune system fights disease itself. We are our own physicians. Problems occur only when the body is under stress.

In order to be self-healing, both body and mind must be healthy, balanced, and well-nourished. That is why almost all forms of natural healing focus on proper nourishment through eating a balanced diet, cleansing toxins that have accumulated in the body, balancing the flow of energy through the body, and reducing levels of stress in your life. In natural healing, drugs, surgery, and harmful substances are never used on the body.

When you visit a practitioner of natural medicine, you will probably have a consultation. Here you will notice the difference from orthodox medicine. The consultation may take longer than a usual doctor's appointment, and the doctor will be interested to know about your whole lifestyle. Your emotional state as well as your physical state will be discussed.

Both naturopath and orthodox doctor will regard missed periods, problems with skin and hair, and so on as symptoms. The orthodox doctor, however, will directly attack what is causing the problem and try to correct it with medication, but a naturopath recognizes that no drug can be given for an unhealthy lifestyle. He or she will suggest that your symptoms are your body's way of way of telling you that you need to make a change in lifestyle and diet. Recommendations will be given about how you can restore you body to good health, such as taking dietary supplements or herbal remedies.

If you think that the treatment is too costly it probably is, so shop around until you find something you can afford or learn about alternative medicine methods yourself. There are many lively and informative books available on the market that can give you the knowledge you require. Do be very careful, though. Just because natural medicine says it is natural does not always mean it is good for you. Many natural therapies are available that are not backed by proper research and do not have proper labeling. Be wary of exaggerated miracle cures that claim to be good for you. Some treatments can cause negative reactions, just as orthodox drugs can. Socrates was killed by hemlock, remember! To be safe make sure you check thoroughly for safety before you take any herbs or dietary supplements or have physical therapy.

RETRAINING THE MIND AND EMOTIONS

It is only in recent times that we in the West have considered the treatment of mind, body, and spirit in isolation from one another. In alternative medicine, these divisions have never existed.

Having a peaceful mind-set can influence your body. We have seen how stress and inner turmoil will aggravate androgen disorder because of the effect stress hormones have on the sex hormones, blood sugar levels, and skin blood flow.

Stress and how we react to it is individual, but we do know that when we are under stress our hormone levels, including the level of androgen, shoot up to deal with the stress. If stress is continuous over too long a period, androgen problems are likely to increase and your condition will worsen. There are many ways to combat stress and soothe the mind, and by so doing to enhance the control and management of androgen-related problems. The following are some of the therapies that have been found to be useful for women suffering from hormonal imbalance.

Autogenics

Autogenic training is a Westernized form of meditation that includes the technique of autosuggestion. It involves both mind and body. The belief is that self-hypnosis can modify the body's natural self-regulatory mechanisms, including the hormonal system. Autogenics involves a set of six specific mental exercises that are repeated when stressful situations arise.

Biofeedback

Biofeedback is a method of recording and monitoring your own responses to stress with special equipment. You are taught how to recognize stress when it happens and how to relax and deal with it. Research has shown that biofeedback can improve circulation and general health. For women with androgen disorder and high stress levels it may be helpful.

Counseling

Counseling is also a means of helping you deal with stress. It will help you understand yourself better and empower you to understand more about your symptoms and how best to deal with them.

Hypnotherapy

Hypnotherapy or hypnosis is a well-established practice that has been shown to help people suffering from stress and anxiety. A hypnotherapist can help you deal with stress and show you how to relax.

Meditation

Meditation is an age-old practice for dealing with tension and stress. The idea is to clear your mind of all troubling thoughts.

The simplest way to do this is to replace those thoughts with something calming or one simple word, such as *peace*, which is repeated over and over again. Meditation is not as easy as it may appear, and to really reap the benefits it is best to learn the practice from a trained teacher.

Relaxation Techniques

Some researchers claim that hormonal dysfunction can be eased with relaxation techniques. Relaxation tries to encourage a deep sense of calm and well-being. Even if the symptoms of your androgen disorder are nor relieved, relaxation can help you reduce stress and improve the quality of your life. Relaxation techniques include listening to music or relaxation tapes, taking a hot bath, and meditating.

Visualization

Visualization is a technique in which you create feelings of health and well-being in your mind. You focus on your hormonal levels and correct the imbalance in your mind. The technique has had some success among cancer patients.

THERAPIES APPLIED TO THE BODY

Physical therapies claim to improve your physical condition, but in many cases they mainly promote a sense of well-being and wholeness—there is a huge overlap here with therapies that focus on the mind and emotions. If physical therapies do bring about any changes in your androgen levels and you are taking hormonal therapy from your doctor, you may need to discuss with him or her some changes in your medication. The following are some therapies that can help you manage androgen disorder most effectively.

Acupuncture and Chinese Medicine

Chinese doctors use herbs and acupuncture as part of an elaborate philosophy that is completely different from that of Western medicine. A doctor will diagnose your condition by looking at your tongue, face, hands, and feet and will counsel you and offer dietary advice. Always the aim is to restore the yin/yang balance between mind and body.

Chinese doctors have always taken problems with a woman's reproductive cycle very seriously. It is thought that the health of a woman's reproductive system is crucial to her overall sense of well-being. If periods are irregular, this indicates that her body is in a state of imbalance. A skilled practitioner will prescribe herbal remedies, recommend changes in diet, and perhaps perform acupuncture.

The aim of acupuncture is to restore the balance of *qi*, meaning energy or life force, in the body and boost parts of the body considered weak. Traditional Chinese practice views the body as a balance between yin (negative) and yang (positive); they are the two complementary qualities of this energy force.

According to the Chinese, *qi* runs through the body underneath the skin like a network. Disharmony and disease follow when this flow is blocked. The reason for the fine needles inserted in acupuncture is to unblock the energy and restore the life force. Among Western practitioners, acupuncture is not a well-known treatment for androgen disorder, but some acupuncturists do use it to treat the condition. The theory is that any kind of hormonal imbalance indicates a blockage of energy flow in the body that needs to be unblocked.

Acupressure

Acupressure is based on the same principles as acupuncture. It is acupuncture without the needles. There are a number of variations, and perhaps the best known is shiatsu. *Shiatsu* is Japanese for finger pressure, and just like in acupuncture, the principles are based on the flow of the life force through the body. Acupressure can stimulate the circulation and possibly the hormonal system.

Ayurvedic Medicine

The Ayurvedic system and yoga techniques are concerned with seven chakras or energy points on the body and the connections between them.

This is one of the main forms of traditional medicine in India. The system is part of a wider philosophy of life known as *ayurveda,* which means the science of life. Like the Chinese, traditional Indian practitioners believe that when the body's energy flow is distorted or imbalanced, the body will suffer with disease and the mind with anxiety. Emphasis is placed on diet, nutrition, lifestyle, environment, and emotions. Herbal and mineral preparations are used to correct hormonal imbalance, and treatment of androgen disorder relies heavily on changing lifestyle and diet.

Aromatherapy

Aromatherapy is the therapeutic use of essential oils that are highly concentrated substances distilled from aromatic herbs, flowers, and trees. They are chemically complex and have hormone-like properties; in addition, they contain vitamins, minerals, and natural antiseptics. Documented use of some of these dates back thousands of years; the ancient Egyptians and then the Greeks used them, and many of their uses have been scientifically tested. Essential oils, when breathed in, send a direct message to the brain, where they can affect the endocrine and hormonal systems via the hypothalamus, particularly relevant for androgen-related disorders. The oils can also affect you through your skin if used in massage, compress, or bath. Tiny molecules of oil pass through the skin and reach the blood and lymph, where they are carried to where they are needed.

There are over forty different oils to choose from; you can either obtain a custom-made blend from a professional aroma-therapist or learn about the practice yourself.

Massaging the abdomen with melissa oil or lavender may help irregular periods. For heavy bleeding, rose oil is recommended, and for painful bleeding marjoram oil. Jasmine oil may be helpful too for any period problems.

For stress, mood swings, and bloating, evening primrose oil may help. Orange blossom for stress and lemon for poor circulation and high blood pressure would benefit those who suffer from diabetes and androgen disorder. Frankincense and tea tree oil can be used for skin problems and lavender to calm and soothe.

Flower Remedies

Flower remedies are used to treat stress and depression. The remedies address both psychological and physical issues and are made from the flowers of wild plants and bushes and trees. There is no scientific evidence to prove that these remedies work, but many people swear by their therapeutic effect.

Homeopathy

The homeopathic principle was invented in 1790 by Samuel Hahnemann. He saw in his medical practice that accepted treatments of his time, such as bloodletting and the use of strong drugs, weakened the body. Homeopaths advocate the use of very small doses of medicine. The solution is then diluted and shaken. Homeopaths believe that the more a medicine is diluted, the more potent the result. The idea is to stimulate the patient's immune system and defense capacity, their overall resistance. Finding the precise individual substance required is the art of homeopathy, but other factors such as stress management and exercise are included in the treatment, which takes into account both body and mind.

Some homeopaths claim that hormonal problems in women can be treated with homeopathic remedies. Graphites or Actaea is often recommended for irregular periods, for instance. Although remedies are available over the counter, you should always consult with a qualified practitioner when taking homeopathic remedies for something as serious as androgen disorder. They tend not to work unless tailored to your individual needs. Always consult your doctor if you are taking homeopathic treatment alongside hormonal therapy.

Hydrotherapy

Hydrotherapy refers to any form of therapy that uses water, including swimming as a means to reduce stress.

Massage

Massage is perhaps the oldest and most influential therapy of touch. It is believed to be very effective in dealing with stress, improving the circulation, and encouraging the body to get rid of waste.

Reflexology

Reflexologists believe that areas on the feet correspond to different organs and parts of the body. Basically, your foot is a map to your body, and therapists believe that by applying pressure to these areas, energy channels are unblocked and restored. With androgen disorder a reflexologist would concentrate on the areas of your foot that correspond to the endocrine glands. Massage would concentrate on your big toe for the pituitary gland and the middle part on the inside of your foot for your adrenal gland.

Nutritional Therapy

Nutritional therapists believe that food is the fundamental factor that causes hormonal imbalance in women. Androgen disorders can improve or deteriorate according to your diet.

A balanced diet will be recommended, and food to which there is an allergic reaction will be eliminated, as will foods that deplete the body of the nutrients it needs. Various vitamin and mineral supplements will be suggested; nutrients and supplements to support your adrenal gland especially will be recommended. Important nutrients for the adrenal gland are vitamin C, vitamin B6, zinc, magnesium, and pantothenic acid. All these nutrients play a crucial role in the health of the adrenal glands as well as the manufacture of adrenal hormones. Evidence suggests that during times of stress, the levels of these nutrients in the adrenals can plummet. For the health of the reproductive organs and to alleviate menstrual and fertility problems, vitamin C, vitamin E, zinc, and selenium will be recommended (see chapter 6 for more diet recommendations).

According to Dr. Michael T. Murray (*Stress, Anxiety, and Insomnia*, p.73), "The adrenal glands can be supported by eating a high potassium diet along with taking nutritional supplements, adrenal extracts and plant based medicines like ginseng." Murray recommends a high-potassium diet as one of the best ways to maintain adrenal function. Fruit and vegetables are rich food sources. He also suggests taking an additional 100mg daily of pantothenic acid, vitamin C, B6, zinc, and magnesium.

Various measures such as taking warm sitz baths, and using clay compresses or caster oil packs on your lower abdomen may also be recommended to stimulate your body's circulation and the endocrine system.

Medical Herbalism

Medical herbalists use plants to treat and prevent disease. Medical herbalists treat the whole person and aim to restore the balance of your body by enabling it with its own healing powers. Treatment will probably also include advice about diet and lifestyle. Herbalism is a serious and refined therapy, and an herbalist must be thoroughly trained to use herbs, which can be potent and at times dangerous. Seek advice from your doctor before you attempt an herbal prescription. Herbal treatments for androgen disorder might include herbs that support adrenal function, such as the ginsengs. Both Chinese ginseng and Siberian ginseng exert beneficial effects on adrenal function and enhance resistance to stress. For irregular menses, herbs recommended include garden rue, spiked aloes, and wild hyssop.

Yoga

Yoga is a system of spiritual, mental, and physical training that originated in India. Yoga therapy promotes the body's own natural healing resources using a holistic approach: a combination of simple postures and breathing and relaxation exercises are taught to promote better mental, physical, and emotional function. Yoga is especially helpful for women with diabetes and/or androgen disorder.

WHAT WE CAN LEARN
FROM ALTERNATIVE MEDICINE

There is much to learn from the approach of alternative practitioners. If you have a hormonal problem you will be treated as a whole person—mind, body, and spirit—and as a result you will be more likely to come to a greater understanding of your body and yourself. You will be encouraged to listen to your body, follow your intuition, and reconnect with your emotions, because if the mind and body are happy and nourished your chances of being healthy increase significantly.

Listening to Your Body

Many women with androgen disorders have somewhere along the line lost touch with their body's needs, stopped paying attention to how their body feels, and ignored the signals their body is sending. Too many times the need to eat, the need to rest, the need to relax, or the need to cry has been suppressed or denied.

Learning to listen to your body may take some getting used to, but in time you will begin to sense when it is sending you messages. Try to listen. If it hurts, stop. If you are tired, rest. If you are hungry or thirsty, eat and drink. If you are full, stop eating. If you feel happy, smile. If you feel sad, cry.

Following Your Intuition

According to Candice Pert, a research professor at Georgetown University Medical center and author of *The Molecules of Emotion*, the immune system, the brain, and most of the organs in the body share molecules. These molecules go back and forth from the brain to the organs and from one organ to the other.

Brain researchers like Pert are discovering a biological reason why intuition can alert us to health problems. When an organ is ill, it signals the brain, and this information reaches the conscious mind and becomes intuition. Intuition then becomes our body's way of saying "I need help."

Women in general tend to ignore, dismiss, or simply miss the signals the body is trying to send them. Women with androgen disorders are no exception. Many know deep down that something is wrong but don't seek advice or treatment. When they find out later that something really was wrong, they are often angry that they did not follow their intuition in the first place.

But how can you be sure there really is something wrong and you are not just being a hypochondriac?

The more in touch you are with your body, the better you will be able to recognize true distress signals. There are ways to help you know your body better and improve your intuition, including imagery, relaxation, and yoga.

Reconnecting with Your Emotions

Many of us find it hard to understand or feel our emotions properly. Emotions are important because they help us experience life more fully. It is not always easy to trust our emotions; sometimes they seem so illogical, and we have been conditioned to delay or deny their expression. Yet the very nature of emotions is to be illogical. Sometimes, for instance, our body just needs to cry or to be angry. Instead of questioning and denying, we should simply allow ourselves to feel what our body wants us to feel.

We may be frightened of negative emotions, but the expression of our emotions, including the so-called negative ones, such as anger, fear, and sadness, will lead to improved physical and mental health. This is not to say that we need to act on them all the time, but we should acknowledge that these emotions exist in order to alert us to areas of discomfort in ourselves. When these emotions are not expressed, they cause even greater stress. When they are bottled up, they affect our whole body, especially the immune system, because we are not allowing ourselves to feel or act as we should. Our emotions are messages that come from our inner wisdom. If they are not worked through, the biochemical effect of suppressed emotions on our immune system will cause physical problems.

Scientists are beginning to understand why crying has a soothing effect. It appears that crying is the body's way of washing out stress hormones. So when people say they are "crying it out," this is literally what they are doing. Stress is linked to increased risk of poor health, and since women cry more often than men, this could be one of the reasons we live longer.

Crying and laughing, feeling and expressing our emotions is the only real way we have to acknowledge that our life matters to us. Feeling our emotions shows us how important our life is to us, and how important it should be to those around us. Sometimes these emotions will cause us pain and distress, but negative emotions also signal the need for some kind of change in our lives. They require us to act, to change the situation that is causing distress, to rebel against what we see as an injustice, to move on with our lives. Negative emotions are not bad emotions, but are necessary for us to grow and develop.

A doctor may help you correct the hormonal imbalance in your body, but ultimately the health of your body, your mind, and your emotions lies in your hands. This is where alternative medical practices may help you come to an understanding that you—and not somebody or something else—are in control of your life.

If you suffer from some of the unpleasant symptoms associated with androgen disorder, you can make healthy life choices. You can improve the quality of your life.

Conclusion

Integrating the Benefits of Both Masculine and Feminine in Your Life

M en and women are different physically. This is empha-
sized in the delivery room, when the doctor pro-
nounces whether the baby is a boy or a girl. Bone
structures in men and women are different. Our heads are shorter
than men's, as are our legs. Our hips are broader, our backsides
will never be as lean, and many of our internal organs are larger.
We have a different chemical balance in our bodies, and while
hormones in men are secreted at a fairly steady rate, ours are of a
cyclic nature. Our basal metabolism is lower than men's, meaning that we can't eat as many doughnuts without wearing them
around our hips. We also have fewer red blood cells and a more
rapid heartbeat, and we live longer.

What makes us different? Until recently, hormones and their
glands were at the forefront of medical research in sexual difference.
Ever since hormones were officially discovered at the beginning of
the nineteenth century, they spearheaded research in this area. It

was believed that there were separate female and male hormones and glands and that this is what defined masculinity and femininity. It was believed that these hormones and glands explained not only physical but behavioral differences. Sexual difference was hormonally determined. It was not long before a two-sex model emerged:

- Men (masculinity): aggressive, independent, unemotional, objective, dominant, competitive, logical/rational, adventurous, decisive, self-confident, ambitious, worldly, leaders, assertive, analytical, strong, sexual, knowledgeable, physical, successful, good in mathematics and science, and the reverse of the feminine characteristics listed below.

- Women (femininity): emotional, sensitive, expressive, aware of others' feelings, tactful, gentle, security-oriented, quiet, nurturing, tender, cooperative, interested in pleasing others, interdependent, sympathetic, helpful, warm, interested in personal appearance and beauty, intuitive, focused on home and family, sensual, good at art and literature, and the reverse of the masculine characteristics listed above.

But then, into this world of cozy sexual stereotyping walked the scientist Bernard Zondek. In 1934, Zondek reported that large amounts of estrogen were present in stallions, traditional emblems of masculinity. The medical and scientific world was forced to reconsider its position regarding hormones. Further studies showed this was also true for humans, not just horses. Not only were there female hormones found in men, but there were male hormones found in women. According to this new account, men and women are not complete opposites at all; instead, different amounts of both "male" and "female" hormones make a person either a man or a woman. Gradually, the traditional two-sex model is fading away.

We now know that men and women, as well as being different, have striking similarities. There really is no such thing as a "male" or a "female" hormone. Despite this, however, traditional views of sex roles still portray the sexes as being as psychologically different as we are physically different. This out-of-date cultural construct lingers on and continues to frustrate and restrict our self-expression. It may even go some way toward explaining the neglect of conditions like androgen disorder. A woman with excess androgens reminds us that men and women may not be quite as different as we would like to believe. The presence of a woman with a medical condition that highlights the masculine potential of her body threatens to destroy all that we have been conditioned to believe about male and female stereotypes.

Learning about the presence of male hormone in a woman's body can give us great insight into what constitutes our true nature. We learn that to be fully healthy we need a balance of both "male" and "female" hormones in our body. There is a small but significant amount of "male" hormone in women and a small but significant amount of "female" hormone in men. Without the presence in our bodies of the hormone of the opposite sex, our sexual development would be incomplete. In order to become whole and be healthy, we need a male hormone. Apparent opposites must be reconciled. We need the masculine, just as the masculine needs the feminine, to function optimally. In our lives we need to learn to integrate the benefits of both masculine and feminine.

The medical term *androgen* might make some of us think of the word *androgyny*. There are many misconceptions about what androgyny means. Many think that it implies the masculinization of women, or the absence of any sex-role definition, that it is somehow associated with homosexuality, bisexuality, physical hermaphroditism, or the loss of sexual identity. All these ideas are wrong. Androgyny comes from the Greek words for man (*andro*) and woman (*gyne*), and it refers to the relatively equal development and flexible integration of both the traditionally

labeled masculine and the traditionally labeled feminine characteristics in one individual of either sex. In its purest sense,
androgyny symbolizes the fully integrated human personality in
which both masculine and feminine forces or energies interact.

In the United Kingdom, plans have been revealed for the
Millennium Dome statue. It will be a reclining man and woman
joined at the hip. The body, represented as a single form composed
of elements of both female and male, is contemplating the future.
The statue symbolizes the androgynous ideal of human complete-
ness and the idea that in our contemporary culture neither sex can
afford to lose touch with either side of our human possibilities.

As women of the twenty-first century, perhaps our greatest
challenge will be to embrace the masculine in our nature in a way
that acknowledges our uniqueness as women. Only when we can
integrate the benefits of female and male qualities in our lives,
only when we can grow out of male-female conditioning and definition by preconceived standards, can we finally be both
uniquely female and complete as human beings.

If you think you have an androgen disorder, I hope this book will
have explained the disorder clearly to you, reassured you that you
are not alone, and encouraged you to seek advice and treatment,
if you are not doing so already.

Having a little too much male hormone is nothing you
should be embarrassed about. Every woman has a certain amount
of androgen. You are not unnatural or losing your femininity. All
of us have both male and female hormones in our bodies—you
just have a little more than usual.

Remember that even if your symptoms are very mild, you
should still see a doctor. Androgen disorders sometimes take years
to manifest fully. They are far easier to treat at this early stage
before you develop serious health complications, such as heart
disease or cancer. Don't think that matters concerning appearance don't merit medical attention, either. They do. Appearance

affects your sense of self-worth. How you feel about yourself is a vital part of good health; a state of good health involves not only your body but also your thoughts and emotions. Feeling good about how you look does matter.

If you are reaching menopause and are androgen-deficient, I hope this book will have helped you make an informed decision about whether or not you wish to have androgen replacement therapy at menopause. Menopause is an exciting and challenging time in a woman's life, and if androgen therapy can give you renewed energy, surely it is worth serious discussion with your doctor.

And, finally, if you don't have an androgen disorder, I hope this book will have shed some light on the role male hormones play in your life. These neglected hormones are crucial to our sense of well-being. They add zest to our lives. Their presence in our bodies teaches us a vital truth about ourselves and human nature. Not only do "male" and "female" hormones coexist within each one of us, but they also work together to function effectively. The two sets of hormones need each other. There is balance and cooperation between the two.

The innate wisdom of our body shows us the way forward into the twenty-first century: balance and cooperation between the sexes, speaking less in terms of mankind and womankind and more in terms of humankind.

Resources

HORMONE TEST KITS

Aeron Life Cycles Laboratories
1933 Davis Street, Suite 310
San Leandro, CA 94577
Tel: 800-631-7900
Fax: 510-729-0383
Aeron Life Cycles is a well-established hormone research unit. It
has recently developed individual patient saliva test kits to measure salivary levels of testosterone, progesterone, estrogen, and
cortisol. You can order saliva kits by phone or fax.

Diagnos-Techs, Inc.
6620 S. 192nd Place, J-104
Kent, WA 98032
Tel: 800-878-3787
Saliva tests can be ordered from this lab.

Meridian Valley Clinical Laboratories
515 West Harrison
Kent, WA 98032

Tel: 800-234-6825
Twenty-four hour urine tests for steroid hormones, including DHEA.

ORGANIZATIONS THAT OFFER ADVICE REGARDING ANDROGEN-RELATED SYMPTOMS

Acne Support Group
Dr. Tony Chu
P.O. Box 230
Hayes, Middlesex
UN4 OUT
United Kingdom
Tel: 011-44-181-561-6868

American Diabetes Association
1660 Duke Street
Alexandria, VA 22314
Tel: 703-549-1500

The American Fertility Society
2140 Eleventh Avenue South, Suite 200
Birmingham, AL 35205-2800
Tel: 205-933-8494

American Hair Loss Council
401 N. Michigan
Chicago, IL 60611
Tel: 800-274-8717

Menstrual Health Foundation
104 Petaluma Avenue
Sebastopol, CA 95472
Tel: 707-829-2744

Resolve Inc. for Women (National HQ)
1310 Broadway
Somerville, MA 02144-1731
Infertility hotline: 617-623-0744

PROFESSIONAL ORGANIZATIONS THAT MIGHT PROVIDE INFORMATION FOR SUFFERERS

American Academy of Dermatology
930 North Meacham Road
Schaumburg, IL 60173
Tel: 708-330-0230

Association of Reproductive Health Professionals
2401 Pennsylvania Avenue, NW, Suite 350
Washington DC 20037-1718

The Endocrine Society
9650 Rockville Pike
Bethesda, MD 20814-3998
Tel: 301-571-1800

International Guild of Professional Electrologists
Professional Building, Suite B
High Point, NC 27262
Tel: 919-841-6631

International Society of Gynecological Endocrinology
8, Avenue Don Boaco
1150 Brussels
Belgium
Tel: 02-771-95-98-771-96-45

National Adrenal Diseases Foundation—NADF
505 Northern Boulevard, Suite 200
Great Neck, NY 10021
Tel: 516-481-4992

National Organization of Rare Disorders—NORD
100 Route 37, P.O. Box 8923
New Fairfield, CT 06812-1783

Society of Clinical and Medical Electrologists
132 Great Road, Suite 22
Stow, MA 01775
Tel: 508-461-0313

ADDICTIVE BEHAVIOR

American Psychological Association
750 First Street, NE
Washington, DC 20002
Tel: 202-336-5500

Anorexia Nervosa and Associated Disorders—
    National Association—ANAD
P.O. Box 7
Highland Park, IL 60035
Tel: 312-831-3438

The Anxiety Disorders Association of America
6000 Executive Boulevard, Dept. A
Rockville, MD 20852-3081
Tel: 301-231-9350

Depression Awareness, Recognition and Treatment (D/ART)
6001 Executive Boulevard, Room 8184 MSC 9663

Bethesda, MD 20892-9663
Tel: 800-421-4211

National Depressive Association
53 West Jackson Boulevard, Room 618
Chicago, IL 60604
Tel: 800-826-3662

PERIMENOPAUSE AND MENOPAUSE

A Friend Indeed: Newsletter for Women in the Prime of Life
Box 515 Place Du Parc Station
Montreal, Quebec
Canada H2W 2P1
Tel: 514-843-5730

American Menopause Foundation, Inc.
The Empire State Building
350 Fifth Avenue, Suite 2822
New York, NY 10118
Tel: 212-714-2398

Menopause News
2074 Union Street
San Francisco, CA 94123
Tel: 800-241-6366

North American Menopause Society
c/o Dept. of OB/GYN
University Hospitals of Cleveland
2074 Abington Road
Cleveland, OH 44106
Tel: 216-844-3334

Power Surge
Web site: http://members.aol.com/dearest/intro.htm

INFORMATION ON ALTERNATIVE/
NATURAL THERAPIES

The American Association of Naturopathic Physicians
2366 East Lake Avenue, Suite 322
Seattle, WA 98102
Tel: 206-328-8510

American College for Advancement in Medicine
23121 Verdug Drive, Suite 204
Laguna Hills, CA 92653
Tel: 800-532-3688
Offers advice on natural hormone replacement.

Association of Holistic Healing Centers
109 Holly Crescent, Suite 201
Virginia Beach, VA 23451
Tel: 804-422-9022

Dr. Christiane Northrup's Health Wisdom for Women
7811 Montrose Road
Potomac, MD 20854
Tel: 800-804-0935
Monthly newsletter.

The Health Resource Newsletter
209 Katherine Drive
Conway, AR 72032
Tel: 501-329-5272
Information on conventional and alternative treatments.

Nutrition Action Newsletter
CSPI
1875 Connecticut Avenue, Suite 300
Washington, DC 20009

Uni Key Health Systems
P.O. Box 7168
Bozeman, MT 59771
Tel: 800-888-4353
Distributes dietary supplements, including adrenal gland support formula.

Women's International Pharmacy
5708 Monona Drive
Madison, WI 53719-3152
Tel: 800-279-5708
Natural hormone treatment.

GENERAL WOMEN'S HEALTH

Harvard Women's Health Watch
P.O. Box 420234
Palm Cast, FL 32142-0234
Women's health newsletter.

HER Place: Health Enhancement and Renewal for Women Inc.
2700 Tibbets Drive, Suite 100
Bedford, TX 76022
Tel: 817-355-8008

Melpomene Foundation
Women's Health and Fitness Issues
Tel: 612-642-1951

Women's Health Access
Women's Health America
P.O. Box 9690
Madison, WI 53715
Tel: 608-833-9102
Bimonthly newsletter on a wide range of women's health topics.

Suggested Reading

Benyo, Richard. *The Exercise Fix: How the Aerobic Athlete's Compulsive Need for the Next Workout Is Self-Destructive.* New York: Leisure Press, 1990.

Borysenko, Joan. *Minding the Body, Mending the Mind.* New York: Bantam, 1987.

———. *A Woman's Book of Life.* New York: Riverhead, 1996.

Burton Goldberg Group. *Alternative Medicine: The Definitive Guide.* Puyallup, WA: Future Medicine Publishing, Inc., 1993.

Chernin, Kim. *The Hungry Self: Women, Eating, and Identity.* New York: Harper Perennial, 1994.

Cheung, Theresa. *A Break in Your Cycle: The Medical and Emotional Cause and Effects of Amenorrhea.* New York: John Wiley and Sons, 1998.

Chihal, Jane, and S. London. "Menstrual Cycle Disorders." *Obstetrics and Gynecology Clinics of North America* 17, no. 2 (June 1990).

Chopra, Deepak. *Quantum Healing.* New York: Bantam, 1989.

Collinge, William. *The American Holistic Health Association Complete Guide to Alternative Medicine.* New York: Warner Books, 1987.

Crapo, Lawrence. *Hormones: The Messengers of Life.* Stanford, CA: The Portable Stanford Alumni Association, 1985.

Cutler, Winifred, and C. R. Garcia. *Menopause: A Guide for Women and the Men Who Love Them.* New York: Norton, 1992.

Dabbs, Jr., James M. "Salivary Testosterone Measurements: Reliability Across Hours, Days and Weeks." *Psychology and Behavior* 48 (1990): 83–86.

———. "Salivary Testosterone Measurements: Collecting, Storing and Mailing Saliva Samples." *Psychology and Behavior* 49 (1991): 815—17.

———. "Salivary Testosterone Measurements in Behavioral Studies." In *Saliva as a Diagnostic Field*, ed. D. Malamund and L. Tabak. Annals of the New York Academy of Sciences, 1993: 177—83.

Day, John. *The Diabetes Handbook*. London: British Diabetic Association, 1986.

Dickey, Richard P. *Managing Contraceptive Pill Patients*. Durant, OK: Essential Medical Information Systems, 1993.

Diethrich, Edward B., and C. Cohan. *Women and Heart Disease: What You Can Do to Stop the Number One Killer of American Women*. New York: Times Books, 1992.

Dreher, Henry, and A. Domar. *Healing Mind, Healthy Woman*. New York: Henry Holt, 1996.

Edwards, C. R. W. *Integrated Clinical Science: Endocrinology*. London: William Heinemann Medical Books Ltd., 1986.

Fausto-Sterling, Anne. *Myths of Gender: Biological Theories About Men and Women*. New York: Basic Books, 1985.

Ferber, Jane, and S. Levert. *A Woman Doctor's Guide to Depression: Essential Facts and Up-to-the-Minute Information on Diagnosis, Treatment and Recovery*. New York: Lowenstein Associates, 1997.

Ford, Gillian. *What's Wrong with My Hormones?* St. Louis, MO: Desmond Ford Publications, 1992.

———. *Listening to Your Hormones*. Rocklin, CA: Prima, 1995.

Franklin, Robert R., and Dorothy Kay Brockman. *In Pursuit of Fertility: A Fertility Expert Tells You How to Get Pregnant*. New York: Henry Holt, 1995.

Gittleman, Ann Louise. *Before the Change: Taking Charge of Your Perimenopause*. San Francisco: HarperSanFrancisco, 1998.

Gravelle, Karen. *The Period Book: Everything You Don't Want to Know but Need to Ask*. New York: Walker and Co., 1996.

Hartog, M. *Endocrinology*. Boston: Blackwell Scientific Publications, 1987.

Hetland, M., J. Haarbo, C. Christiansen, and T. Larsen. "Running Induces Menstrual Disturbances." *American Journal of Medicine* 7, no. 1 (1995): 53–60.

Hogg, Anne. "Breaking the Cycle: Sufferers of Amenorrhea Now Have Better Treatment Options." *American Fitness* 15, no. 4 (July–August 1997): 30.

Hudson, Tori. "Androgens and Women's Health." *Women's Health Update*. http://www.thorne.com/townsend/mar/wns_update.html.

Jansen, Robert. *Overcoming Infertility: A Compassionate Resource for Getting Pregnant*. New York: W. H. Freeman, 1997.

John, F., and D. Ebling. "The Biology of Hair." *Dermatology Clinics* 5 (1987).

Johnson, S. *From Housewife to Heretic*. Garden City, NJ: Doubleday, 1981.

———. *Going out of Our Minds: The Metaphysics of Liberation*. Watsonville, CA: Crossing, 1987.

Jovanovic, L., and G. J. Subak-Sharpe. *Hormones: The Women's Answerbook*. New York: Ballantine, 1992.

Jubiz, W. *Endocrinology: A Logical Approach for Physicians*. 2d ed. New York: McGraw-Hill, 1985.

Kelly, L., J. Jansen, G. Chapler, and J. Cook. *Precocious Puberty: Information for Families*. Iowa City, IA: University of Iowa, 1990.

Kingsley, Philip. *The Complete Hair Book: The Ultimate Guide to Your Hair's Health and Beauty*. New York: Grossnet and Dunlap, 1979.

Kolodny, Nancy. *When Food's a Foe: How You Can Confront and Conquer Your Eating Disorders*. New York: Little Brown, 1992.

Lee, John R. and Virginia L. Hopkins. *What Your Doctor May Not Tell You About Menopause*. New York: Warner, 1996.

Legro, R. S. "The Genetics of Polycystic Ovary Syndrome." (Proceedings of a Symposium: An NICHD Conference: Androgens and Women's Health.) *The American Journal of Medicine* 98, no. 1A (1995): 9s–16s.

Levine, Barbara. *Your Body Believes Every Word You Say*. Boulder Creek, CA: Aslan Publishing, 1991.

Lukas, Scott E. *Steroids*. Springfield, NJ: Enslow Press, 1994.

McGarth, Ellen. *When Feeling Bad Is Good*. New York: Henry Holt, 1992.

Medvei, V. C. *A History of Endocrinology*. Lancaster, England: MTP Press, 1982.

Monahan, William. *Eat for Health*. Tiburon, CA: Kramer, 1989.

Mondimore, Francis M. *Depression: The Mood Disease*. Baltimore, MD: Johns Hopkins Press, 1990.

Morgan, Brian. *Hormones: How they Affect Behavior, Metabolism, Growth, Development and Relationships*. New York: Berkeley Publishing Group, 1989.

Murray, Michael T. *Stress, Anxiety, and Insomnia: How You Can Benefit from Diet, Vitamins, Minerals, Herbs and Exercise*. Rocklin, CA: Prima, 1995.

Nachtigall, Lilla, and J. Rattner. *Estrogen: The Facts Can Change Your Life*. New York: Harper & Row, 1986.

Northrup, Christiane. *Women's Bodies, Women's Wisdom: Creating Physical and Emotional Health and Healing*. New York: Bantam, 1995.

Olds, Linda E. *Fully Human: How Everyone Can Integrate the Benefits of Masculine and Feminine Sex Roles.* Englewood Cliffs, NJ: Prentice-Hall, 1981.

Orbach, Susie. *Hunger Strike: The Anorectic's Struggle as a Metaphor for Our Age.* New York: W. W. Norton, 1986.

Ornish, Dean. *Eat More, Weigh Less.* New York: HarperCollins, 1993.

———. *Love and Survival: The Scientific Basis for the Healing Power of Intimacy.* New York: HarperCollins, 1998.

Pert, Candice. *The Molecules of Emotion.* New York: Scribner, 1997.

Piel Cook, Ellen. *Psychological Androgyny.* New York: Elsevier Science, General Psychology Series, 1985.

Pleck, J. *The Myth of Masculinity.* Boston: Massachusetts Institute of Technology, 1981.

Rako, Susan. *The Hormone of Desire: The Truth About Sexuality, Menopause and Testosterone.* New York: Harmony, Random House, 1996.

Redmond, Geoffrey. *Androgen Disorders.* Austin, TX: Raven Books, 1985.

———. *The Good News About Women's Hormones: Complete Information and Proven Solutions for the Most Common Female Hormone Problems.* New York: Warner Books, 1995.

Redmond, R. *Lipids and Women's Health.* New York: Springer Verlag, 1991

Reichman, J. "Testosterone . . . for Women?" *American Health for Women* (October 1998): 43.

Reiser, P., and M. Underwood. *Growing Children.* San Francisco, CA: Genentech, 1991.

Rittmaster, R. S. "Clinical Relevance of Testosterone and Dihydrostestosterone Metabolism in Women." (Proceedings of a Symposium: An NICHD Conference: Androgens and Women's Health.) *The American Journal of Medicine* 98, no. 1A (1995): 17s–26s.

Roth, Geneen. *Feeding the Hungry Heart: The Experience of Compulsive Eating.* New York: N.A.L Books, 1982.

Schaef, A. W. *Women's Reality.* New York: Harper & Row, 1982.

Scrambler, Annette. *Menstrual Disorders: The Experience of Illness.* London: Tavistock, 1993.

Seaman, Barbara. *Women and the Crisis in Sex Hormones.* New York: Rawson Associates, 1977.

Shealy, Norman, and C. Myss. *The Creation of Health.* Walpole, NH: Stillpoint Publishing, 1987.

Sheeley, Gail. *Menopause: The Silent Passage.* New York: Pocket Books, 1993.

Shuttle, P., and R. Redgrove. *The Wise Wound: Myths, Realities and Meanings of Menstruation*. New York: Bantam, 1990.

Singer, June. *Androgyny: The Opposites Within*. Gloucester, MA: Sigo Press, 1989.

Skolnick, Andrew A. "'Female Athlete Triad' Risk for Women." *Journal of the American Medicine Association* 270, no. 8 (August 25, 1993): 921–923.

Steven, Catherine. *Diabetes: A Comprehensive Guide to Effective Treatment*. Boston, MA: Element Books, 1995.

Strauss, R. H., M. T. Ligget, and R. R. Lanese. "Anabolic Steroids Use and Perceived Effects in Ten Weight-Trained Women Athletes. *Journal of the American Medicine Association* 253 (1985): 2871–2873.

Taylor, William N. *Anabolic Steroids and the Athlete*. Jefferson, NC: McFarland, 1982.

Vincent, L. M. *Competing with the Sylph: Dancers and the Pursuit of the Ideal Body Form*. Kansas, MO: Andrews and McMeel, 1979.

Vliet, Elizabeth Lee. *Screaming to Be Heard: Hormonal Connections Women Suspect and Doctors Ignore*. New York: M. Evans, 1995.

Waterhouse, Debra. *Outsmarting the Female Fat Cell: The First Weight-Control Program Designed Specifically for Women*. New York: Hyperion, 1993.

Weil, Andrew. *Natural Health, Natural Medicine*. Boston: Houghton Mifflin, 1990.

———. *Understanding Conventional and Alternative Medicine*. Boston: Houghton Mifflin, 1995.

Williams, M. H. *Beyond Training: How Athletes Enhance Performance Legally and Illegally*. Leisure Press, 1989.

Yen, S. C., and Robert B. Jaffe. *Reproductive Endocrinology: Physiology, Pathophysiology, and Clinical Management*. Philadelphia, PA: WB Saunders Company, 1991.

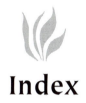

Index

HOW WOMEN CAN *FINALLY* STOP SMOKING
by Robert C. Klesges, Ph.D., and Margaret DeBon, M.S.

This guide addresses the special needs women have when trying to quit smoking. Based on Memphis State University's highly acclaimed smoking-cessation program, this book reveals that what works for men does not necessarily work for women. Women's bodies react to nicotine differently, so withdrawal symptoms are more severe; and when they stop smoking, women gain weight more easily than men do. A handy pull-out card with a stop-smoking checklist and self-monitoring diary show a woman the times of day when she is most likely to want a cigarette, allowing her to prepare herself to resist the urge.

192 pages ... Paperback $11.95

WOMEN'S CANCERS: How to Prevent Them, How to Treat Them, How to Beat Them *by* Kerry McGinn & Pamela Haylock   *Revised 2nd edition*

Women's Cancers is the first book to focus specifically on the four cancers — breast, cervical, ovarian, and uterine — that affect women most, offering the latest information. The book approaches the subject in a clear style, and describes successful prevention, detection, and cancer treatments in detail.

512 pages ... 68 illus. ... Paperback $19.95 ... Hard cover $29.95

HER HEALTHY HEART: A Woman's Guide to Preventing and Reversing Heart Disease Naturally
by Linda Ojeda, Ph.D.

Heart disease is the #1 killer of women ages 44 to 65, yet up until now most of the research and attention has been given to men. This book fills this gap by addressing the unique aspects of heart disease in women and natural ways to combat it. Dr. Linda Ojeda explains how women can prevent heart disease whether or not they take hormone replacement therapy (HRT). She also provides detailed information on how women can reduce their risk of heart disease by making changes in diet, increasing physical activity, and managing stress.

352 pages ... 7 illus. ... Paperback $14.95

Prices subject to change

ORDER FORM

10% DISCOUNT on orders of $50 or more —
20% DISCOUNT on orders of $150 or more —
30% DISCOUNT on orders of $500 or more —
On cost of books for fully prepaid orders

NAME

ADDRESS

CITY/STATE   ZIP/POSTCODE

PHONE   COUNTRY (outside U.S.)

TITLE	QTY	PRICE	TOTAL
Androgen Disorders in Women (paperback)	@	$13.95	
Once a Month (paperback)	@	$15.95	

Prices subject to change without notice

Please list other titles below:

	@	$	
	@	$	
	@	$	
	@	$	
	@	$	
	@	$	
	@	$	
	@	$	

Shipping Costs:
First book: $3.00 by book post ($4.50 by UPS, Priority Mail, or to ship outside the U.S.)
Each additional book: $1.00
For rush orders and bulk shipments call us at (800) 266-5592

TOTAL	
Less discount @____%	(_____)
TOTAL COST OF BOOKS	
Calif. residents add sales tax	
Shipping & handling	
TOTAL ENCLOSED	

Please pay in U.S. funds only

❑ Check ❑ Money Order ❑ Visa ❑ Mastercard ❑ Discover

Card # _____ Exp date _____

Signature _____

Complete and mail to:

Hunter House Inc., Publishers
PO Box 2914, Alameda CA 94501-0914
Orders: 1-800-266-5592   email: ordering@hunterhouse.com
Phone (510) 865-5282 Fax (510) 865-4295

❑ Check here to receive our book catalog

ADW 6/99